Staying Healthy
Throughout Your Years

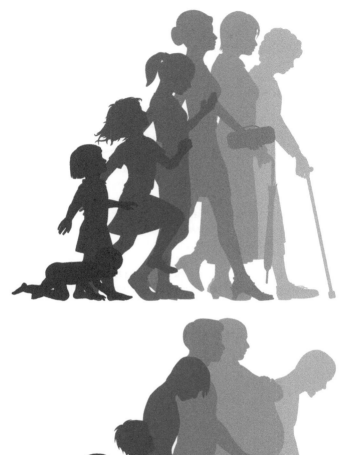

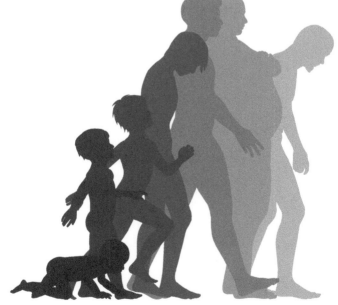

It is Loving to be Born, Great to be Nurtured
A Challenge to Continue on, and an Honor to Grow Old.

Edmund A. Cruz

AuthorHouse™
1663 Liberty Drive
Bloomington, IN 47403
www.authorhouse.com
Phone: 1 (833) 262-8899

Because of the dynamic nature of the Internet, any web addresses or links contained in this book may have changed
since publication and may no longer be valid. The views expressed in this work are solely those of the author and do
not necessarily reflect the views of the publisher, and the publisher hereby disclaims any responsibility for them.

Any people depicted in stock imagery provided by Getty Images are models,
and such images are being used for illustrative purposes only.
Certain stock imagery © Getty Images.

This book is printed on acid-free paper.

ISBN: 978-1-7283-6415-5 (sc)
978-1-7283-6417-9 (hc)
978-1-7283-6416-2 (e)

Library of Congress Control Number: 2020913357

Print information available on the last page.

Published by AuthorHouse 08/04/2020

authorHOUSE

Staying Healthy
Throughout Your Years

By
Edmund A. Cruz

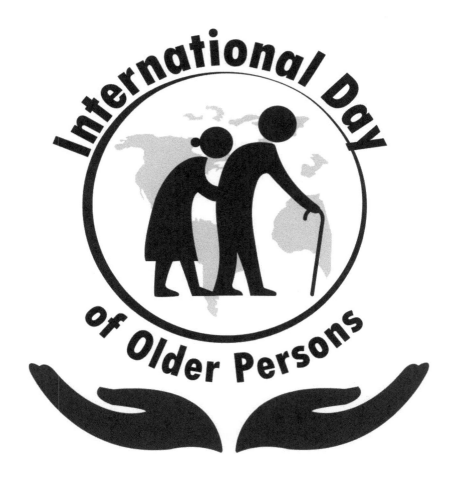

About the Author

Edmund A. Cruz is a natural for writing about health and physical fitness in all its forms and remains physically active. He is a Registered Professional Nurse with a B.A., B.S. and an M.S. with numerous other certificates and certifications in the field of medicine and emergency care. Mr. Cruz worked in various psychiatric hospitals throughout the State of New York for the State of New York. He has worked at Saint Vincent's Hospital Emergency Room and in the Intensive Care Units, Beth Israel Hospital Emergency Room, Booth Memorial Medical Hospital Intensive Care Units and Emergency Room, and in Manhattan Eye, Ear, and Nose Hospital Emergency Room. He also worked as an EMT/Paramedic for Saint Vincent's Hospital. His skills range from a Critical Trauma Care Nurse, an Instructor in Prehospital Pediatric Care, an Instructor in EMS/EMT/Paramedic which are all courses certified by the Department of Health and Emergency Medical Services of the City of New York. Mr. Cruz has an Honorable Discharge from the United States Air Force and later enlisted in the United States Army Reserves of which he has retired from as a Lieutenant Colonel. In the Army, he has taken the Army Master Fitness Course and was in charge of the physical training program for his commander. Mr. Cruz is a Graduate of the Command and General Staff College of the Army. He has taken many health-related courses and they all were licensed by the State of New York Education Department. Mr. Cruz has also taken a number of physical training instructor courses, such as, American Academy of Personal Training Course and the National Federation of Professional Trainers Course. As you can see, Mr. Cruz is very well versed to write about health issues and has written other books on Health maintenance and Physical Fitness topics.

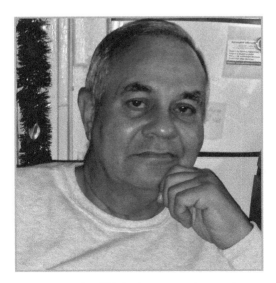

How you take life's journey is up to you

Edmund A. Cruz

In the beginning of life's aging journey, we do not really become older, we actually mature. This maturing continues until we reach the highest level of our body's perfection or completeness and then we return to life's beginning.

Edmund A. Cruz

Acknowledgement

I would like to thank my wonderful wife for her patience, her editing, her advice, and her share love and dedication in helping me with all my books and writings. She is my inspiration and the heart of my life and my writings.

Edmund A. Cruz

It is the purpose of this writer that this book be used to help the younger generation better understand the elder population, their struggles, and desires to remain part of the contributing element to the whole of our society. It is to convey information on establishing and maintaining the health of all of us but mainly those that are more senior then most. Becoming of a senior age will come to all in time but it should not come as a surprise that separates us from the youngest or older population or them from the rest of society. Our seniors should be a source of inspiration, information, understanding, resource, and for all to look towards for advice, wisdom, help, and comfort in times of need. Our seniors should be treated with respect, honor, and most of all love. This writing was done for all these reasons and to try and protect one of the most venerable, valuable, and most esteemed members of our society; our senior citizens.

The material in this script are those of the author and are the latest information at the time of publishing. Guidelines concerning practices and procedures, rules and regulations governing the writing of this information may and can change. It is up to the reader to review, challenge, understand, and familiarize themselves with local, state, and federal regulations in their area. The author and publisher of this book disclaim any liability resulting in direct or indirect suggestions and theories, errors or omissions, and misunderstandings that have or may be made in the writings of this material. This material is not to diagnosis, treat, or cure any ailment, disease, or untoward illnesses. It is basic information related to all as well as the senior population that may be of interest to that and all demographics and genders. A professional review in the field of the area of interest needed in these chapters should be sort out for classification, clarification, information, and further understanding of the material. No part of this writing is to be reproduced or transmitted in any form or by any means without the written permission of the author.

Author of "Staying Healthy: Throughout Your Years" is Edmund A. Cruz

Illustrations in this book are from Shutterstock.com

All proceeds from this book will be donated to The AARP Foundation

Why This Book

Before deciding to write this book, I was writing another book called "The Beginning, The Journey, and the Final Destination of Man" this stopped after I was involved in a car accident that crushed many of my fingers on my left hand. I was rushed to the nearest hospital that had an orthopedist surgeon and after a little hospital shuffling, I was eventually operated on, admitted, and then discharged in three days after surgery. I became very depressed and for a long period of time gave up on writing and many other things. When the bandages were removed after one month and when I saw the horrible conditions of my fingers and how badly they are mangled and how deformed they were, it made me even more melancholy. I was literally embarrassed to go outside and when I had to, I wore gloves. You see, I am a very active person, I go to the gym three to four times a week and I pride myself on my physical appearance. Now I am deformed and very conscious of how my hand looks and how others see my deformed hand. What bothers me the most is that I felt defenseless in protecting my family, friends and myself. I have always considered myself the protector, and now, I am not so sure. I started physical therapy approximately two in a half months after my surgeon took out the pins from my finger. The surgeon said that I can resume a gradual return to my normal routine but what the heck does that mean? For the next three and a half months of physical therapy and going three times a week, I struggled to bring my fingers back to some assemblance of normalcy. During my time in physical therapy, I had the great occasion and honor to meet Dr. Nilesh Soni, DPT, GCS, MS, MA, PT, who is the owner of the Physical Therapy Center. We became friends and talked about many things especially about geriatric concerns and health care which he truly believes, aspires to, and practices in his profession. It just so happens that during our conversation I happen to tell him that I have written books on health-related topics and found out that he read some of my books and he liked the way I wrote. Dr. Soni suggested that I should write a book on the elder population: their medical concerns, on elder injuries, treatments and care, the elder social issues that befalls them, and some of the mental concerns and changes that may be a part of the growing old process. He specifically asked me to write it like my other books in an easy to read and understanding manner in which I have written my other books. After a month or so, I took his advice and gathered information for the writing of this text. My depression is still present but has lifted a great deal and I feel a lot better about myself. I have even gone outdoors more and I have found the will and strength to go back to the gym. Dear friend, I hope I did some justice in this book for you and all who read this book. To all, have a long and healthy life from me and Dr. Nilesh Soni.

Preamble

There is one thing that life will bestow on all of us and that is the aging process. We are all going to get old, this is inevitable but what is not so clear is that we all have the means to grow old and age with the least amount of discomfort and the most grace as humanly allowed. Your genes may hold the genetic code as to aspects of your biological make-up but you hold the trump card as to the quality of life you wish to lead. As it stands now in the U.S.A., the average expected human survival age is anywhere from 77 to 79 for men and 80 to 84 for females take or give a year. This really is not adequate. The human body is capable of living a much longer lifespan. In order to find out what makes the human body work and how to optimize life's fullest potentials as to its pathophysiology one must find out "what does age mean and what causes this process." We now have the understanding and means to determine the why of the aging process. Some of the key questions that need to be answered in the why quest is do we have to age and if so, what happens to our body during this aging journey, more importantly, can we stop or slow the aging journey process down. The answer to the second part is; Yes. There are a number of theories as to what happens as we age and grow older and why this aging process actually happens; some of these main theories are **The Gene Theory,** the **Damage DNA Theory,** and the **Damage Mitochondria Theory.** In "The Gene Theory" the question remains does the gene already have our life expectancy prerecorded? If that is the case, can the advent of modern science in some way advance or change this DNA genealogical process. Can we alter the **apoptosis** (programmed cell death) and slow it down to improve and maintain the tissues homeostasis and increasing the DNA program to a program for living longer than the present gene has encoded? In the Damage DNA Theory, we will look at what is causing this death of cells to happen, is this death of cells caused by damage to our DNA and our neurons and if so is the precursor or cause due to free radicals usurping and making the DNA weak or is it breaking it down and causing the cells to become old too soon, thus causing the DNA cell to no longer function properly and eventually die? If this is the case, is there a way to slow down or even reverse the production of this free radical constructs in our body's? In the Damage Mitochondria Theory, is exercise good since mitochondria produces energy via ATP for movement and exercise and since exercise breaks down the mitochondria making more free radicals once the energy is used up? Does this mean that there are more free radicals floating around in our body after a heavy workout? To be honest, it doesn't matter which theory is the correct one or if all three theories are working in sync combination. All of us have a say in how well we care for our health in this respect. The DNA controls only a third percent of how our body's longevity code and this goes for how well we maintain our health. Again, only a third of this is part of the DNA/biological function. The other seventy percent is controlled by the human factor; **YOU.** This means that you control most of the quality of life you will live. It is you that determines the direction your body is going to take, that is, either increasing or decreasing the overall accumulated damage to your cell's DNA. You have the power to either speed up or slow down the aging process. Yes, we can slow down the aging process and that means by changing some of the habits one has developed over the years. This also means adding new habits to your lifestyle with some modifications to one's diet, energy expenditure, and weight management. When it comes to the aging processes, you control the medical, physical, neurocognitive, and environmental attachments and early cognition. Using sound judgment will help in treating and getting through these changes to your life with the best possible outcome. Understanding basic anatomy and physiology of the body and how the body's chemistry is involved in our health and in controlling and/or eliminating impurities including free radicals. How does free radical chemicals break down DNA cells? These are all questions that need some clarification and explanation and a rational working plan. What's important to understand is what foods should you eat, how often you should eat them, how much one should eat as well as when is the best time of the day you should eat. Are vitamin supplements needed and if so, are they affective? As we grow older, are their nutritional supplements that are especially important for the aging process that are needed to maintain good health. How does all this play such a dynamic role in the production of the byproduct made by foods, the effects it has on the body and the production of free radical formation. The one question that still remains is, what the heck is a free radical and how does it actually damage DNA? Is a healthy and proper diet really able to reduce free radical formation and can antioxidants really work in reducing damages caused by free radicals and increasing the life of the DNA cell? What role does exercise play in health and longevity? Does exercise have any role at all in maintaining a healthy body? Is exercise a real player in increasing or decreasing free radicals in the body and will it increase one's longevity or reduce it? When it comes to protecting the senior citizen, what laws are there and when does elder mishandling become a problem. How can an older person seek assistance when it comes to medical help and health care? Is there a means to plan and prepare for a medical emergency and is there a format to follow if the need arises that a medical emergency response is necessary? How does one access this emergency help? These and many other questions will be answered in this short but important text on **"Staying Healthy: Throughout Your Years."**

For the Reader

I just want you to know that you and I are going to die. In fact, we are all going to die and with proper care and good health as we age, the assassin is going to be **Time.** Time is the mother of birth and the limits of existence. It waits for no one and does not discriminate against race or creed, poor or rich, woman, man or any animal, and it does not care about the color of a person's skin. Time has a beginning and an end; it never goes backwards only forwards and it is in sole control over life. It has no friends or enemies and follows one path which is just a one-way trip. How you take that path or journey through life is all up to you. Now that we have settled that and got that out of our way let's get to life and to living. We are all here on earth on borrowed time and how we use this borrowed time will be determined by the choices we make and this will determine how well and how long we will live on this borrowed time. It is obvious that in order to live or survive on this planet we have to adapt to earth and its elements. Earth does not want us to live here so we have to change with earth on a continuous cycle of survival. Albeit, we cannot just allow earth to dictate life's cycle upon us or except the cycles of aging that the earth throws at us and we cannot allow earth to take its toll upon our body's. No, it is up to each and every one of us to find ways to stretch this life out and to do this in a way that maintains our health in mind, body, and in a soulful spiritual manner. Realizing that no one's tomorrows are guaranteed, there are some predictors of a heathier and more fruitful existence on earth. Here's what we can do today to get some extra tomorrows. There are certain ways of living that we have discovered throughout the centuries which can extend the life expectancy of mankind. First, we must distinguish between normal aging patterns and separate this from the problematic aging patterns or risk factors and the fragilities of aging which may be a part of some aging processes. This may require some understanding of the anatomy and physiology of the human body, how and why it works, what alerts the brain to tell the muscles or organs how to function, what makes the mind aware of things, the cognitive processes that remembers time and events, and understands concepts. What part of the brain receives and what part forwards information to the many cells in the body for them to work, in other words what triggers the cells in our body to perform, and how is all this put together so it works for you as a coordinated mind and body harmonization. It is also important to understand what causes the cells of the body to breakdown and age. Is it possible to slow this process down and if so how? We are all going to age **period** but with a good diet, proper sleep, reduction of stressors, and some exercise along the line one can achieve a healthier life. This book is not meant to teach you how to become old, that will come with time, it is meant to try and explain how to live and grow old with pride and dignity with as much health and grace as humanly possible. It does not matter when you start your health endeavors, I'm here to remind you to just start. Eleanor Roosevelt once said, "Yesterday is history, tomorrow is a mystery, but today is a gift that's why it's called – present." Keep your body fit, nourished, and young in body, mind, and spirit, that's what real living is all about. You only have this one shell of a body to live in for a short period of time so live in it proudly with all the love you can give it until time calls us back to the beginning.

Contents

Chapter 1

What do We Mean by "Staying Healthy?"

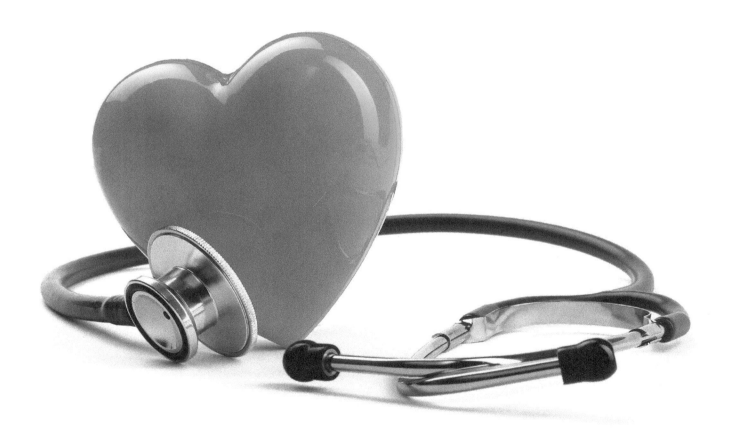

Contents in Chapter 1

What do We Mean by "Staying Healthy"?

In human biology there is a continuous balancing act of **homeostatic** changes going on within the body. When this **homeostasis** starts to slow down and/or fail, it is defined as the aging process which is the amount of time during which a person lives. Humans, as with most living things, depend on this highly balance state between the internal biological balance and the external environmental balance conditions one goes through in life. This life balancing actually continues in a forward direction. It depends on how one follows this path in life with these changes and alterations in the paths processes as to how well we live our lives. In many ways this stumbling forward makes life interesting throughout this journey as we age. Most of these factors we journey through depend on the kind of choices we make and it is these choices which can and will compound all other internal and external factors that can either add to or subtract from a person's quality of life and longevity. Life is a fickle thing and the human body is just its shell or chapel that we have to use during this process in these life decisions. This body or shell must be cared for and carried forward throughout this journey of human existence. One cannot live without this shell so we must be proud of and respectful to this shell for its use and keep this shell healthy and maintaining this chapel or shell with good health and strength during one's use of its biological existence. This is the only shell you're going to have and live in so it is important for you to take care of it for as long as you have use of it; and so, the meaning of this title **"Staying Healthy: Throughout Your Years."**

How Long Will I Live?

It has been determined that a person's **genetic** code dictates their life's expectancy or span of time on earth; at least this is what most people think. Actually, this is partly true, the life expectancy is based on the **gene** but it is also based on many other factors. In the United States the chronological age of 65 is classified as the so-called elder population. I totally disagree with this assessment. There is no definitive borderline of age and though by using 65 may be good practice because of Medicare options, insurance plans, or retirement options it is just wrong. People are stigmatized by this chronological calculation. Only the human body and its physiological functions can truly define what old age is. Believe it or not time ages all of us differently. Have you ever noticed that some 40ish or 50ish year old's function physically and mentally like older or younger people than their chronological age and that some 20-year old's have the wisdom of a much more mature individual? Chronologically, older age groups do not necessarily equate to physical, biological, or psychological points of view other than a point of reference or opinion that one chooses. This is due to more than just the gene but how society frames and uses it in regard to how one actually lives. In fact, the gene accounts for approximately 30 percent of the physical, biological, and mental developmental functions and the longevity expectations that an individual will survive pass the age of 70 or 80. To be quite honest, over the past 80 years the life expectancy throughout the world has doubled. With this increase, we can expect to live well pass 70 barring any environmental or unforeseeable events. This extended **longevity** (the extent of one's life) is due to the combination and contributions of the genes and modernization of society, the advances in medical innervations as in new vaccinations for diseases, development of antibiotics and discoveries in better sanitation methods, the control and prevention of infantile illnesses, and the many other health related advances brought about through science in all fields. What follows is that one can have a coded gene disorders that can contribute to health-related conditions and still live a very long life. It is very likely some of these older individuals have a gene related form of chronic ailment maybe even more than one ailment that needs ongoing treatment or hospitalization but regardless of this coded gene life is then extended due to this modernization. There is a rise in the elder population due to all this innovation. This can be seen when one accounts for the increase in the population of older adults seeking medical intervention in doctor's offices, clinics, and in various other health care facilities and in medical specialty areas, such as, emergency rooms, and in the number of hospital admissions throughout the country as well as in the number of hospital discharge referrals for continuation of treatment modalities and follow-up care.

Gene Theory

Living a long life is great but this is not what we all really want to know is it. What we really want to know is how well one's health would be with this added or extended life line. That is the big mystery. Would we be subjected to these common age-related diseases like cancer, unhealthy bones, cardiovascular disease, vision related problems, and/or **dementia?** What we do know at this time is that making life time choices at the earliest possible age plays an important role in future lifestyle of health related conditions of an individual. This, in no way, means that starting a healthy lifestyle at a later age would not contribute to a longer and healthier life outlook. Lifestyle choices like a good diet, routine exercise, refraining from smoking and reducing alcoholic consumption can play a great part in determining how long and how well one lives and also how well one's health is setting itself up to be. Healthy habits are a great determiner of what to expect and it is this waiting time that is a factor in determining one's long life's journey that will later affect your entire life going into your golden years. There is a way one can determine if they have a good possibility of a long-life cycle and that is by researching the family tree. By reviewing the history of your family's health and life span, certain traits can reveal health related conditions and illnesses as-well-as a possible added bonus of one's expected lifeline may be seen and/or followed. Research into analyzing the **genome** (gene cell) one can determine genetic markers in your **DNA (Deoxyribonucleic acid)** that will contribute in some degree to one's inherent life expectancy. This also means that one may inherit predispositions involving conditions to diseases, such as, weaknesses or strengths and illnesses past down by your ancestors. These predisposing conditions are within the matrix of one's DNA but does not necessarily mean an offspring will inherit that specific genome marker that causes, let's say, obesity or long life.

Sometimes these genome markers require a trigger or an event to activate them. Specific genes may jump two generations before it is activated or triggered. So, just because grandma lived to 95 years of age does not automatically grant the offspring this trait even though it is in the gene.

What Role Does the DNA Play in Longevity?

When talking about DNA molecules, we are talking about a **chromosome** with all or part of its genome or genetic material of an organism and in this case the organism is homo-sapiens. Within the chromosome or DNA molecule, it is important to understand that the DNA has specific variations which can either contribute to a longer life or shorten it through a disease progression or by genetic markers within the complex genetic modifications. These diseases processes in the modifications to longevity can be **diabetes, cardiovascular disease, dementia or Alzheimer's disease,** bone discrepancies like **osteoporosis,** and **hypertension** to mention a few. Then you have your **centenarians** which have **exceptional longevity (EL)** of 100 and more. These centenarians have a variation of genetic indicators called **SNPs or single nucleotides polymorphisms** that perhaps were the contributing factor for this long life. To simplify what SNPs are we must first say that this is the most common type of genetic variation in the human body. It is a single DNA called the **nucleotide** which is the building block of the DNA and **RNA (Ribonucleic acid)** and is in the molecules of all living things on earth. There are over 5 million SNPs in the human body and it depends on how they are paired that is associated with the biological diseases one acquires such as diabetes, hypertension, obesity, dementia, etc. It also has an effect on how you tolerate drugs, environmental factors, toxins, and longevity traits. It is this dependence on the complex combination of variances in these nucleotides that determine the biological human condition. Although there have been a lot of research on genetics, scientists feel that they have some understanding and are getting an upper hand. There are just so many other fundamental factors that are involved in the total make-up of the gene and the environment that actually make it difficult to make any sense of what really contributes to a longer and healthier life. Genealogical research continues to study the socioeconomic status, the climate one lives in, the weight and height of a person, even the mate's one chooses may all be a contributing factor in living longer. It is still unclear as to why females, on the average, live about five years longer than males. Each person, male and female, have different life spans with the average for male being 78.93 and female 83.6 as of 2020. When one ponders the question, "how long can humans live" not every molecular geneticist and/or Gerontologist can answer this question because there may be no answer or limitation, at least, no answers to this question at this time. We know that humans have lived to 110 and older, in-fact, in April 2018, Emma Morano passed away at the age of 117. She was the oldest living person at the time. In 1997, Jeanne Calment of France died at the age of 122. Humans that live longer than 110 are referred to as **supercentenarians.** So, to answer this question, "How long will I Live" well, there may be no limitation as to how long humans can live. What is a fact is that you're going to keep getting older until you die: fact! The consensus of opinion is that there is no real age limit in humans. There is no biological reason why humans cannot live to be 150 years old or even older.

What Causes Aging?

We do not know what causes aging but we do know the physiology of aging and the process of becoming old. Just to make it clear, we will just be referring to human beings in regard to knowing the physiology of aging. Cells within our body cease to function and cease dividing which is called cellular **senescence** (the condition or process of deterioration with age). Scientists have a theory that this stated condition is due to what is called **"The Damages Cell Concept."** What is known is that it is the failure of these cells whereby DNA oxidation takes place and accumulates which eventually damages the cells and the DNA. There are three well known concepts: **"The Gene Theory", "The Damaged DNA Theory," and "The Damage Mitochondrial Theory."** In **The Gene Theory** there is a belief that adaptive evolution occurs through the differential survival of competing genes and since inherited information is in the gene which is passed down from one offspring to the other through the DNA it is considered as a natural selection or best of the best of the species that are chosen to continue on. **The Damaged DNA Theory** concept is that aging is the consequence of unrepaired accumulation of damaged and dead cells due to the lack of oxygen and nutrients being blocked by these inactive cells. Although, both mitochondrial and nuclear DNA as well as RNA damage can contribute to this blocked aging process. **The Damage Mitochondrial Theory** has two variables: mitochondrial free-radical and non-free-radical theory of aging (MFRTA). The MFRTA proposes that free-radicals produce ATP and this ATP produces electrons that can escape from the mitochondria and react to water producing reactive-oxygen species (ROS) or free-radicals. ROS can damage macromolecules including lipids, proteins, and DNA which can speed up the process of aging. These damaged DNAs can also cause the progression of a variety of other conditions such as cancers, mutations, and cell repair problems. DNA **methylation** is another way that can change the way the DNA molecules work which can change the activity of the DNA function with the addition of a methyl group that is added to its bands. The RNA is also subjected to damage just like the DNA. Damage to the RNA may cause changes in the activity and the sequence which can act to repress gene transcription (copying) causing neurological disorders such as Alzheimer's disease, **Parkinson's disease,** and dementia. This damage can cause other physiological, psychological, and even neuro/social changes which will slow down or break down cells causing a cascade and eventually failure over time. Some of the physical and mental aging experiences one will journey through as we become older are dependent on your lifestyle choices throughout the years. **Free radicals,** for instance, are responsible for the oxidation of some of the cells. These free radicals are unstable molecules that damage and accelerate the break-down of DNA. Free radicals are also linked to the causes of cancer. Scientists have developed a way to detect this type of damage to the DNA and RNA.

It should be understood that DNA can be damaged by normal wear and tear of the body through time and this time would contribute to cell death. Features, such as, smoking, sedentary life style, alcohol, and even too much sunlight are also factoring in to this cell destruction. Just for information purposes, there is an extreme form of aging that hits the very young that is called **progeria.** This is a severe mutation of the **XPF gene,** a gene involved in the repair of the DNA. This is not the only gene involved in repairing DNA for normal aging but it is being researched and studied to determine what role it plays in the aging process and how it causes progeria. All these causes of aging including oxidation stress, the damage cell concepts, telomere shortening, mutation, aggregation of protein, and free radical theory can be summed up in that it is the progression of all of these expects that are damaging to these cell structures and functions that is seen as the total course of the pathophysiology in the aging process.

DIFFERENCES BETWEEN DNA & RNA

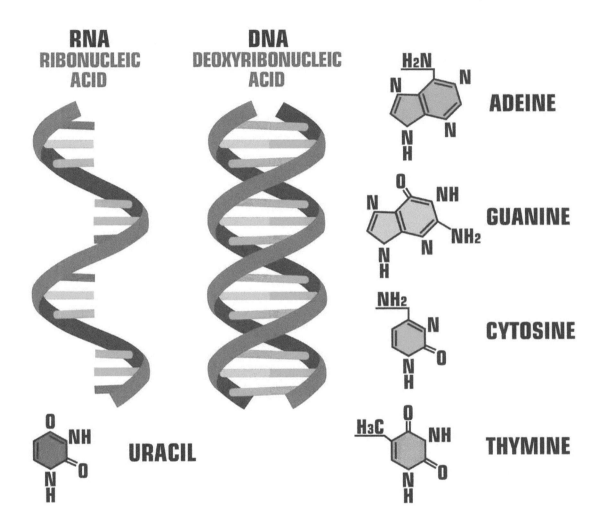

RNA
RIBONUCLEIC ACID

DNA
DEOXYRIBONUCLEIC ACID

ADEINE

GUANINE

CYTOSINE

URACIL

THYMINE

What are Free Radicals?

Free radicals are a chemical species that contain a single unpaired electron in its outer orbit. The body actually needs and uses free radicals to sustain life. Free Radicals come from the foods that we eat, the air we breathe, and are caused by some of the medicines we take. The chemistry in our body breaks down these foods or medicines making free radicals to produce energy for function and these free radicals are necessary in the building up of our immune system. Free radicals also have other essential life supporting requirements for the maintenance of health and the continuation of life. Your body is constantly making free radicals because it is the byproduct of all the chemical processes of metabolisms that builds up and breaks down the cells of the human body. How are free radicals produced? As your body uses oxygen, the oxygen molecule is split and loses an electron which then becomes a single atom. This single atom that is formed has now become an unpaired electron. Electrons do not like to be without a mate or unpaired so it seeks out other electrons and if it finds a free radical it will take it as its paired electron with the atom. This is called **"the oxidation process"** and this pairing may cause damage to the cell, the protein, and the DNA. There is a **nucleus** (DNA) that is also found in the **mitochondria** which is one of the **organelles** in the cells **cytoplasmic body** so when the mitochondria makes energy it creates **ROS or "reaction-oxygen species"** what we now call free radicals that can damage other mitochondrial DNA and make them lose their ability to function causing loss of body energy; More on this later.

FREE RADICAL
AND NORMAL MOLECULE

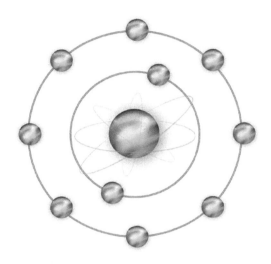

STABLE MOLECULE

FREE RADICAL
MISSING ELECTRON

Mitochondria Scheme

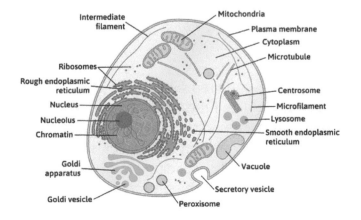

The Human Cell

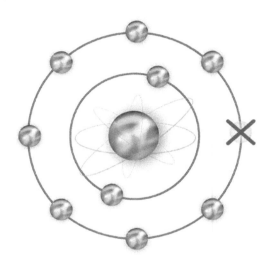

Mitochondrial DNA

Although there is no way of testing for free radicals directly, there is a way of testing and analyzing lipid **peroxidation.** This is an indirect method for testing for free radicals and it is by measuring the oxidative degradation or breakdown of lipids since free radical's steal electrons from the lipid's membrane causing damage to the lipids in the process. The question is "can we slow down or neutralize this free radical damage" the answer is **yes.** There is a number of methods to slow down oxidation and they are by good nutrition, exercise, and building a healthy body.

- **Antioxidants** – are molecules in the foods we eat that prevent free radicals from taking electrons and causing damage. It is a natural substance found in beta-carotene and other carotenoids, lutein's (green leafy vegetables), resveratrol (similar to Vit. E), Vit. C, Vit. E, lycopene (found in tomatoes), selenium, and other phytonutrients.
- **Cells of the body** – is that the body produces its own antioxidants but many times it is insufficient in number to function efficiently on a daily basis with the stressors inflected on it.
- **Exercise** – increases the production of free radicals by using extreme amounts of energy by breaking down the mitochondria and damaging the cells. It is this breaking down and rebuilding of the mitochondria that enhances, strengthens, and improves the antioxidants ability in the body to bond with a single electron.

Immortality and Aging

Yes, there are species that are immortal, such as, bacteria that can reproduce daughter cells, certain plants can clone themselves, and animals in the phylum class that have the ability to regenerate, in-fact, never actually grow old. Four billion years ago, life was formed on earth from the **primordial soup** an inorganic element or compounds of goo that eventually united to an organic compound or the molecules of life.

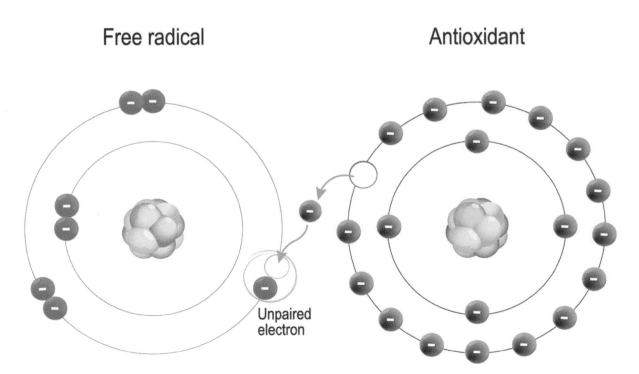

Free radical   Antioxidant

Unpaired electron

This chemical process is called **abiogenesis** or informally – the origin of life on earth. Phylum organisms such as the Cyanobacteria, Prokaryotes, Protozoans, and algae are single celled organisms that are plants and animals that multiply by fission producing daughter cells through a process called **photosynthesis** which means they do not age and are essentially considered immortal. Humans have cells with this ability or potential for immortality: cancer cells for instance, such as, the **HeLa cells** line and specific **stem cells or germ cells** (those producing ova and spermatozoa) have the ability to maintain life as long as they are properly nourished and cared for. **Cloning** of adult cells is the process of reproducing an identical organism or individual either by natural or artificial means. This research is still ongoing. The human liver has the ability to reproduce, repair, and heal itself because it has **telomerases** but for most of the regular cells in a normal human body, they do not have telomerase abilities to heal or replicate cells and so after about 50 to 70 cell divisions the cell dies. We have touched upon DNA's and nucleotide's or SNP (single nucleotide polymorphism) but it is important to know that the base-pairing will determine specific traits on which one would have inherited specific parent traits. **Telomeres** (Greek word meaning "ends") are bodies of DNA nucleotides or proteins that are located at the end of the chromosome which protects the chromosome from shredding or deteriorating. The telomere is like the plastic coatings on a shoe lace. Each time the chromosome replicates the telomeres at the end of a DNA wears away and become shorter until it is used up and once used up the enzyme that duplicated the DNA can no longer be replicated or reproduced because the telomeres are used up: gone.

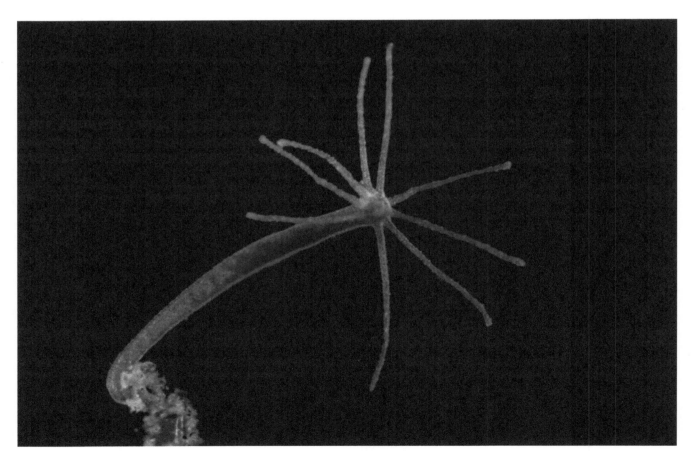

Genus Hydra Species (Phylum Class)

As the telomere's ends are used up, the cell becomes senescence and cannot divide anymore consequently the cell dies. As this process of shortening of chromosomal telomeres continues to happen, you will have damage and death of cells, so goes the process of aging. Much of the cells aging in the human body is caused by the culmination of many other factors four of which are;

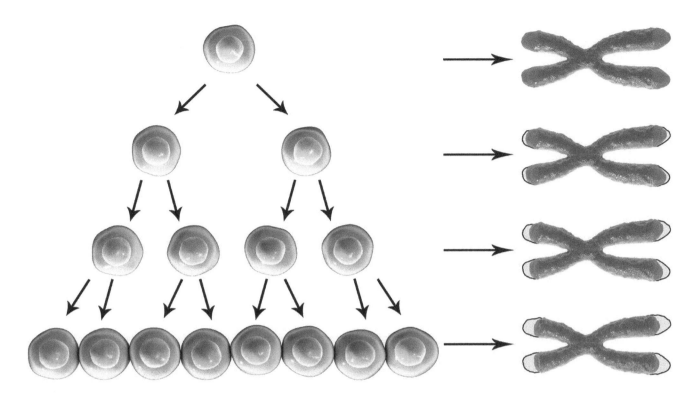

The average cell divides between 50 to 70 times and as the chromosome telomeres get shorter, they cannot duplicate anymore and the cell dies.

Cellular aging which is, as stated above, the number of times your cell replicates which is about 50 to 70 times. This is due to the wearing out and shortening of the telomeres, free radical damage, and other factors,

Metabolic aging is the process of changing foods into energy that the cells need to function. This process of breaking down foods to produce energy for the body results in a byproduct and/ or free radicals which some are needed by the body and is good but in excess free radicals can cause damage to the body over time,

Hormonal aging is the process of metabolism that is due to the continuous changes in hormones throughout our life from childhood to maturity,

Accumulated damage is the total of the above and wear and tear damage of the body's internal environment and that can be caused by external factors that one is continuously exposed to and endures over a lifetime.

As stated, the evolution of sexuality and all that it entails in human reproduction which is said to have started over a billion years ago, provided the means to be able to transfer and/or pass on genetic material to produce a new off-spring and in this way the survival of the species flourished. So ends immortality. Now, as we become older, changes linked to aging start to take place; your cells start to slow down in their division, such as in growth and repair of body cells; a decrease in one's ability to recuperate after an injury, illness or disease will also slows down; eyesight and hearing difficulties develop; tissue pliability which is tone and texture is decreased due to loss of collagen; hormones and gland secretions diminish which causes a cascade of other physical, psychological, and emotional changes as well as bone dyscrasias especially in females; diminished ability to tolerate stresses, a decrease tolerance to drugs and in the inability in fighting diseases; and-so-on-and-so-forth. Welcome to the mortal human condition.

During our life time, the aging process takes on many other more personal forms and characteristics throughout most of our human journey through life. Although mentioned above, a more intimate look into human aging is the development of wrinkles, decline in female fertility and the on-set of menopause, vision declines and the need for reading glasses, graying, thinning and loss of hair, arthritic conditions, adult on-set of osteoporosis diseases arises, hearing and cataract may become part of our living routine, heart and vascular disease may ensue and become major problems. What is the most depressing of the age-related ailment is when neuro-cognitive impairment or dementia rises its ugly head and takes over the one we love and intervenes with the family's core relations. This memory loss is literally the loss of a person's life that was well lived with all thoughts and deeds erased regarding family ideals, values, history, and even survival skills. These starts to change the core family member's essence bringing this particular love one back to a more infantile behavioral dependent state. This is indeed hard on all and is a sad albatross to bear for the remaining love-ones, friends, and caregivers. Breaking it down a little further, aging depends generally on how we take care of ourselves. Remembering that 30 percent of the aging process is related to one's DNA, the remaining 70 percent is controlled by the human factor and not the DNA. That means, the human factor is you; you can control most of who you are and how you will live your life not the DNA.

Aging is not a uniform process, that is, aging effects of the eyes or the skin or the lungs do not all age at the sometime. Your body cells, organs, tissues, and brain, will age at different rates and degrees as well as at different times during this time spent process. Your eyes may age first and glasses may be need to read or you may start losing your hair or graying of the hair may develop early, your equilibrium may be compromised and balance may become a problem first, then in time your breathing may become a problem, etc., etc., and so-on. Yes, time is marching on and aging with it; this **IS** unavoidable. No one is immune to time so everyone will be affected and yes, aging does not discriminate as to race, creed or nationality. Aging affects every cell in the human body eventually in the same way but this process can be slowed down so that you can enjoy the fruits of your labor and live a healthier and longer life. There are many helpful ways and hints which are well known, such as, the five basic group factors; not smoking or drinking alcohol or ceasing these activities, exercising regularly at least three to five times a week for about 20 to 30 minutes even a simple walk is good, obtaining adequate rest and **that means sleep;** having and/or maintaining a good social life which is very important to the mind and the body so keep connected to people; and reduce as much stress factors as one possibly can. Life is not an easy task; it is like a gang of misfits trying to climb Mount Everest with every step being a new challenge. Everyone is learning how to live well every single day and it is this trial and error scenario that we must make the choices in how we should maintain our balance in life. I have always said that the main purpose in life is to live it with dignity and integrity and to be true to your principal values. Benjamin Franklin once said, "We get old too soon and wise too late" so let's reverse Benjamins Franklin's wise wisdom and use it to make smart healthy choices earlier in life to live a better and longer tomorrow.

What is Frailty?

As stated above, as we become older certain risk factors start to appear. These risk factors or time warning signs have been well covered above but many of these adverse or unhealthy signs of the aging sequela are not part of the normal outcome of a life's downward expectation. Declining age does have the characteristics of weight loss, fatigue, reduced activity, and physical weakness. Some accumulation of other medical problems and situations may appear and some may be a part of the normal aging cycle of life. There are other changes that are not part of this normal aging trend. These physical changes are often referred to as the **frailty of age** or **"the geriatric syndrome."** According to the American Geriatric Society of the National Institute on Aging in 2004, "frailty in older adults is a state of increase vulnerability to stressors due to age related decline in physiological reserve across neuromuscular, metabolic, and immune systems." There have been many concepts as to what frailty is and I will just summarize and say 'what the general consensus' is that according to the theory it all comes down to the same thing; the more health related problems an individual has and the older the adult is predicts the frailty of the individual. This frail state on the chronological age is the risk factor itself so the theory goes. According to the common consciences, frailty is associated with aging and cognitive decline, the decrease rate of physicality which goes along with physiological functions, and an increase rate in the risk factors in developing diseases is the criteria. Going further with this type of thinking and so called research, it is claimed that those in a lower educational levels, those that smoke, persons that become or suffer from depression, people in the lowest socioeconomic scale, are unmarried, or are in the Latin/Hispanic or African American race have the highest risk of health related complications that will lead to being physically frail. Some of the health complications associated with this type of thinking in the category of older frail adults are;

- Congestive Heart Failure,
- Diabetes Mellitus,
- Hypertension,
- Peripheral Vascular Disease,
- Brittle Bones Disease Syndrome,
- Dementia.

There was a comparative study conducted by Women's Health and Aging Studies that was done in two parts - 1 and 2 as well as, other studies such as Survey of Health, Aging and Retired in Europe (SHARE) in a three-year study period on men when it came to mortality in regard to robust men or frail men. To their amazement, it was discovered that the men in the frail group had a 2 percent or higher risk of mortality then the more robust healthier men. At this juncture, it is important to go over again the definition of frailty and what is meant by a robust. In a simple way, **frailty** is a quality or state of weakness, disabled, unhealthy individual, and especially the elderly adult person, and the other elder **robust** group having vigor, strength, and good health. These are two opposites, so to what purpose was this time, study, and probably a lot of money spent meant to prove, for me; it was a waste of time and expense not to mention basic logic. It is quite obvious that the frail aged adult would have a higher incident of health-related morbidity and mortality as well as other related ailments in comparison to the less high-risk factors in the healthier more robust older adult. It is also quite obvious that the frail older person would have a less favorable outcome during a surgical procedure with an increased risk of postoperative complications, discharge planning, and follow-up control. These assessments and studies do not mention the environmental impact that may have played a part of the study or its countries of origin that were assessed; was this a worldwide population study or just done under more modern industrial and economically robust sound countries? Realizing that only men were taken into consideration during the study survey, what were the race, ethnic groups, geography, climate, and seasons of the study? This was not recorded in the study that was presented.

Physiological Processes in Aging

Although some pathophysiology was discussed, it is important to go into it in a little more detail. The biological aging process starts from the time of conception and does not end until we have returned to nature. For humans, aging is an ongoing process and this journey continues for all carbon-based organicism's. As infants, we are frail and in need of assistance and are totally dependent on others for needs. As we develop to maturity, we become more and more independent, able to make more rational decisions and choices. These choices produce stresses that will eventually take its toll on the human body and how well we live. This will be governed by the progressive and continuous choices put upon the body causing stresses we must deal with or make and eventually upon how it will weigh in as to how well our cells age. There is an awareness in scientific cycles that the stresses of life can and do make molecular changes in our body and are due to these choices that produce stresses as to how our body regulates the hormones and energy produced in response to the stresses and used by the body. As stated above, these stresses can be internal or external, environmental or socioeconomic to cultural and so on from hard working people to the rich and famous individuals. There is no group not touched by the stresses of the aging process.

After saying this, I do not doubt the frail and even the robust older adult individual will, as time goes by, have anatomical and physiological declines in skeletal bone integrity, muscle function strength changes, endocrine and immune alterations which are the key components of the frail state. The decline in hormones in the body will activate the inflammatory pathways causing molecular variations and chemical instabilities that will alter biological function. One of these endocrine hormones affected is the insulin known as **IGF-1.** This hormone is produced by the liver and plays an important role in childhood development and the **anabolic** (protein synthesis) effects on every cell in the body especially the skeletomuscular systems on growth progression in adults. In older adults, there will be a decrease in this **insulin growth factor (IGF-1)** which will be associated with lower muscle strength and movement or mobility. It is not entirely clear what triggers this degenerative process but poor nutrition, exercise status, age, sex, ethnicity, stress, estrogen, and other bodily functions is physiologically clear. To sum it up in one name, it is called **sarcopenia;** more on this in a later chapter. A gradual decrease in muscle mass and strength will eventually start, which is a normal expectation, around the age range of thirty-to-forty. Sarcopenia is a component of this frailty syndrome and is classified as a disease that affects 10% of the adult population over the age of 50. Other hormones that can and/or may decrease are adrenal androgen **Dehydroepiandrosterone sulfate (DHEA-S),** reproductive hormones estrogen and testosterone, and an increase in **cortisol** levels which will affect your immune system and skeletal muscles system which can contribute to the frail state. Please be aware that there are other physiological and endocrine changes occurring during the this aging progression which are part of the normal adult aging process. It becomes more symptomatic when there are added impairments and specific disease states associated in this process to the aging path which are warning signs for the high risk of adverse health related conditions.

Assessment Tools to Determine States of Frailty

There are many assessments and measuring tools for determining degrees of frailty in older adults that have been developed over the years. Your evaluator may use the **Frail Scale** which is one of the measurement tools used and which is a quick way to determine the human **phenotype** or physical assessment of the frailty condition. This method of frailty testing is recommended by the Geriatric Advisory Panel of the International Academy of Nutrition and Aging and the data gathered was from the Cardiovascular Health Study done in two parts in 1989-1990 and 1992-1993 of women and men 65 years of age and older. They were followed-up for 7 years the first time and 4 years the second time respectively and examined annually and were asked these few questions;

1. Do you find that you're always tired,
2. Do you have problems walking up or down the stairs,
3. When you go out, do you have problems walking one block,
4. How often do you get sick or feel ill,
5. How much weight did you lose in a three-month period,
6. Do you have problems getting out of a chair.

These questions and others will provide a predictable validity for a physical frail state. This test is not a definitive answer to the frail risk assessment test of an adult individual but it can give a reference area to start. There are other frail measuring tools such as weakness of the person's grip strength, poor endurance, walking gate speed and balance while walking, and low activity and energy expenditure in other words, how fast does he/she become tired while performing a task. Finding a clinical syndrome for a frail condition in an older adult requires much more intervention. Other assessments test is the determination of ruling out any other medical or psychological concerns that may influence frailty conditions. Your physician may request laboratory testing which may include routine blood count, metabolic panel workup, test workup, urine test, vitamin B12, Vitamin D, and TSH (Thyroid Stimulating Hormone) testing. All of this should be assessed and evaluated before a determination of a frail diagnosis is made. Once a frail state is determined, there are no real guidelines as to the management of the frail older adult other than providing a safe environment and risk prevention programs governed by providing ongoing medical care as needed. It is important to provide help and assurance that the individual is able to maintain physical activities as well as perform ADL (activities of daily living). Interventions can include adding exercise routines like walking, stationary biking, mild calisthenics, nutritional counselling, and maybe even nutritional supplements as needed.

In summary, we are all going to get old and how we progress from infant, child, and adulthood to old age is up to the individual. Yes, we were born dependent on others and eventually we will all become dependent on others again during this last journey through this twilight of our life's cycle. The majority of us can expect a normal aging process but some will have a more difficult time and so the progression of this frailty of the body and mind and yes, it is looming as we age but it does not have to be the more difficult path, depressing or a debilitating form. We have to think smartly now so that time can be less of a mystery, more healthier, and much brighter. The elder population should not be categorized only by age, race, or socioeconomic status but by the ability to function, to produce, and to contribute to society and that should include friendship, love, and companionship. As we grow older and time moves on, the risk factors are inevitable and become greater with the loss of physical strength and bone density, our senses become less acute especially hearing and balance, as well as, vision, smell, taste, and touch. Movements, balance, and posture become more of a challenge due to the declining inner ear and the eyes and its connections to the brain. Since the human body was never inherently developed for standing up-right on two feet this type of movement becomes a continuous encounter with our internal and external environment and yes, gravity becomes a major challenge and concern. This and our senescence may cause our balance or equilibrium to become problematic and situational leading to falls. Falls occur when the demands of the posture are exceeded and the body is incapable to respond to that demand of gravity. We can choose to maintain good bearing and a healthy lifestyle or squander it away with other less favorable options but that's up to the individual. To this day, there is no known standard for the verdict as to what is a true diagnosis of what constitutes to a frail state in the elder adult. There are many assessment tools that can be used to screen what is considered a frail older adult and one of these methods that are recommended is from the **International and Worldwide Consensus Group** called **The Frail Scale** assessment which states that once one reaches the age of 70 and those older adults with chronic ongoing disease processes or those that lose 5% of body weight in a year should be classified as frail. Personally, this is nonsense! Judging on these bases is an affront to humanity but The Frail Scale at least gives a much sounder foundation for suspecting a frail condition although further test and physical evaluations with psychological profiling is a better prognostication.

Chapter 2

Chemical Aspects of Anatomy and Physiology

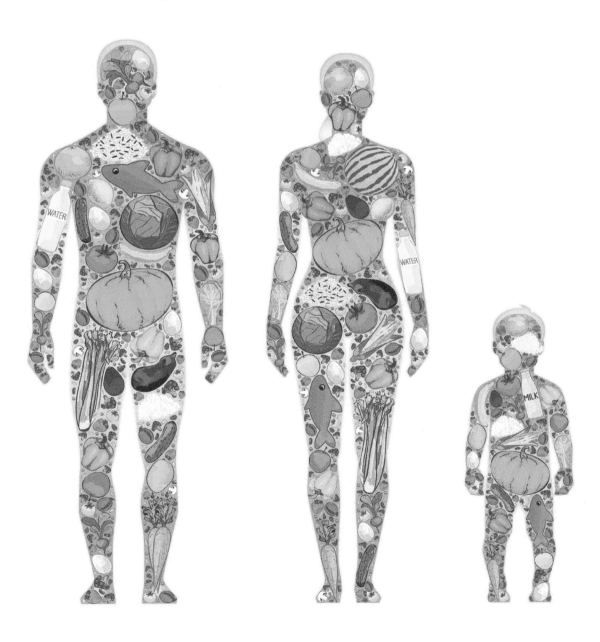

Contents in Chapter 2

Chemical Aspects of Anatomy and Physiology

Learning the basics of the anatomy and physiology especially the building blocks of the human body and how it works is important in better understanding the more delicate details and functions of the aging process. In this and in the following chapters an introduction to the basics of the anatomy and physiology will be presented with the assumption that the reader has had no previous knowledge or study of the human body. This text is geared towards that beginner with the added introduction of the aging process to and for the general population at large. These chapters will cover basic levels of organic chemistry, the musculoskeletal system and joints, and the nervous system. It will also go into some clinical aspects and applications within its specific subject domain with the idea of better understanding of what the aging processes is. Again, this is going to be very brief on the pure basics chemical elements and anatomy and physiology of the human body.

Chemical Elements

The bonding of organic substances depends on the atoms forming a molecule. The atoms are what all elements are composed of while the molecule is the units of its compound. Matter is in all living and non-living things. This matter is in solids, liquids, or gaseous forms. All matter is made up of building units called **chemical elements** which cannot be decomposed by ordinary **chemical reaction** (molecules interacting to form new bonds [more on this later]) and at present there are 106 elements on the **Period Table of Elements** of which 92 come from natural form. Out of these elements 26 are found in the human organism with most found in trace amounts.

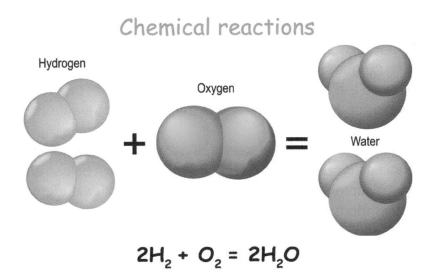

Chemical reactions

Hydrogen

Oxygen

Water

$$2H_2 + O_2 = 2H_2O$$

The Structure of Atoms

To repeat, all matter in the universe is composed of a substance known as elements. An element is composed of atoms which is the smallest part of an element. All atoms consist of two basic parts: the nucleus and the electrons. An element cannot be broken down further without losing the properties of that element. Atoms have positive charged particles called protons (p^+) and negative charged properties called electrons ($e-$). There is a particle called a neutron (n^0) that has no electrical charge. The proton and the neutron separately weigh 1835 times more the electron. The electron surrounds the proton in an orbit and the proton and neutron adhere tightly to each other in the center forming a dense positive charged nucleus of the atom. The electrons spins around the nucleus which is centrally located and comprises most of the atomic mass.

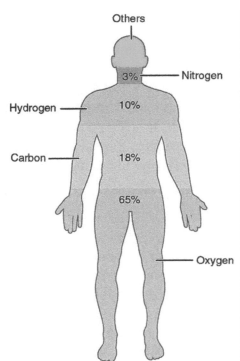

Element	Symbol	Percentage in Body
Oxygen	O	65.0
Carbon	C	18.5
Hydrogen	H	9.5
Nitrogen	N	3.2
Calcium	Ca	1.5
Phosphorus	P	1.0
Potassium	K	0.4
Sulfur	S	0.3
Sodium	Na	0.2
Chlorine	Cl	0.2
Magnesium	Mg	0.1
Trace elements include boron (B), chromium (Cr), cobalt (Co), copper (Cu), fluorine (F), iodine (I), iron (Fe), manganese (Mn), molybdenum (Mo), selenium (Se), silicon (Si), tin (Sn), vanadium (V), and zinc (Zn).		less than 1.0

The **atom number** is the number of protons found in an atom and the **mass number or weight of the atom** is the total number of the protons and the neutrons in the atom. If an atom has 6 protons then the atom number is 6 and the mass number would be 12 as in carbon, in nitrogen the atom number is 7 and the mass number is 14 (remember that protons and neutrons adhere to each other). The diagram below are full stable outer shells of electrons.

The most stable atoms are those that have a full outer shell of electrons like 2 electrons or 8 electrons. Atoms without a full outer shell of electrons will either gain or lose an electron until its outer shell is full again and the atom becomes stable. This is called an **inert element** because there will be no reaction with other atoms. **Oxidation** is when the atom loses an electron and when an atom gains an electron this is called a **reduction.** They often occur together and when they do it is called **oxidation-reduction reaction.** However, when they lose or gain an electron, the atom acquires a charge and becomes **ionized.** It is a positive charge atom if it has an extra proton and negative

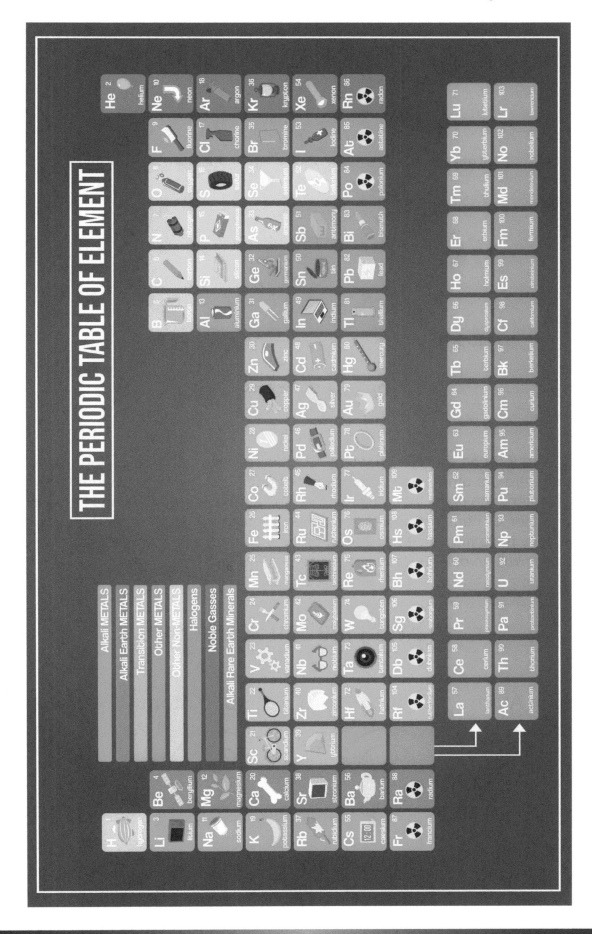

Atom structure

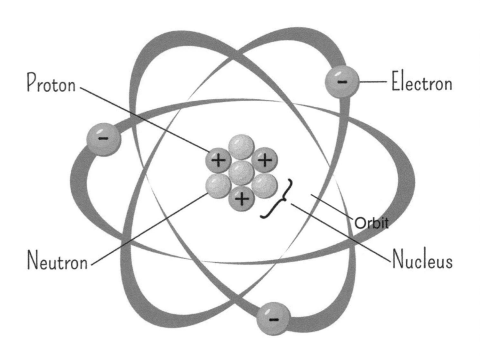

charged atom if it has an extra electron. Sodium, calcium, and potassium are all ionized atoms and there are other ionized atoms in the body that are important for the physiology and the maintenance of life. Atoms that have the same number of protons for each element but the number of neutrons varies are called **isotopes** and although they have variant neutrons, they have the same number of protons so the atom number is the same but the mass number will be different.

Drawing the Simplest Atoms

Hydrogen Atom

$+ = 1$
$- = 1$

Oxygen Atom

$+ = 8$
$- = 8$
$\bigcirc = 8$

Carbon Atom

$+ = 6$
$- = 6$
$\bigcirc = 6$

Nitrogen Atom

$+ = 7$
$- = 7$
$\bigcirc = 7$

$+ =$ proton
$- =$ electron
$\bigcirc =$ neutron

Atoms and Molecules

As atoms breakdown or combine with other atoms, a chemical reaction occurs and a new product with different properties are formed. This chemical reaction is the foundation of all life processes. A molecule is the combination of two or more atoms (chemical reaction) and this combination of atoms can be the same kind as in the hydrogen: H2 molecule or different atoms as in hydrochloric acid molecule: HCl. A **compound** is a substance that can be broken down into two or more different substances by chemical means and these elements are always different. **Chemical bonds** are what hold the elements in a compound together. There are three types of bonds - **ionic bonds, covalent bonds, and hydrogen bonds.**

- ○ **Ionic bonds** – is when the electrons of one atom transfer to a second atom. Each atom has different charges, positive or negative, and is opposite of the other electrons; negative to positive, etc. Example: sodium and chloride or Sodium chloride (NaCl)

- ○ **Covalent bonds** – is when two atoms share one or more electrons. Example carbon and 4 hydrogen atoms or oxygen and hydrogen: water/H20. When a single pair of electrons is shared, the bond is called a **single bond;** when two pairs are shared, it is called a **double bond.**

- ○ **Hydrogen bonds** – is a hydrogen atom covalently bonded to one oxygen atom or one nitrogen atom, but attracted to another oxygen or nitrogen atom. These hydrogen bonds are weak bonds because they cannot bond atoms to molecules and serve as a bridge between two molecules. The hydrogen bond is also known as an **electrostatic bond.** It is part of the DNA and is located between a pair of other atoms and a component of the nucleic acid that holds the double helix together.

An important component of many chemical reactions and the universal solvent for the human body is water. The human body is over 75 percent water and physiologically it participates in most chemical functions.

Chemical Reaction

As we have already stated earlier, a chemical reaction is the making or breaking of bonds between atoms. In a chemical reaction, the total number of atoms remains the same but because they may be rearranged, the molecules are new as well as the properties.

1. **Synthesis Reactions/Anabolism** – is combining two or more atoms, ions, or molecules. This reaction involves the 'forming of new bonds' A and B being the **reactant** and the final substance formed is the **end product.** All synthesis reactions in your body are collectively called anabolic reactions or just **anabolism.** The reaction direction is indicated by the arrow.

to form

A   **+**   **B**   →   **AB**

Atom, ion, or   Atom, ion, or   New
molecule   molecule   molecule

2. **Decomposition Reaction/Catabolism** – means to breakdown into smaller parts and is the reverse of anabolism. In this reaction the bonds are broken. Decompose means to breakdown into small parts.

breaks down into

AB → **A** + **B**

Molecules AB   Atoms, ions, or   Atoms, ions, or
molecules   molecule

Acid, Base, and Salt

An **acid** is defined as a substance that **dissociates** (breaks down or ionizes) into one or more hydrogen ions (H+) and one or more negative ions (**anions**). This chemical action produces an electric charge called **electrolytes.** It is also called a proton (H+) donor when broken down. A **base** may be viewed as a proton acceptor. **Salts** are made up of sodium and chlorine and has a negative charged ion (OH_) and a positive charged ion (H+) and are attracted to each by an **electrostatic force** called an ionic bond. Water breaks down (dissociates) into **cations** (a positive charged ion and anions) which is a basic or base solution called an **alkaline** solution. Salt ions are the source for many essential chemical elements and depending on how much hydrogen ions are released would determine the strength or weakness of the acid.

Acid - base reactions

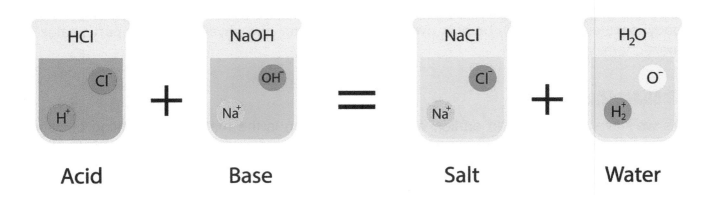

Acid   Base   Salt   Water

The pH Concept

When we measure the **acidity and alkalinity** (acid and base) we use the term **pH** and it refers to the number of hydrogen ion concentration of a substance. When the hydrogen ions and hydroxyl ion (OH-) are equal, the pH is said to be 7.0 (pure water is 7.0). It is important to keep in mind that a solution must be in an aqueous solution to have a pH. Acids have a lower pH and alkaline have a higher pH so a pH below a 7 is an acid because it has more H+ then OH- and a pH with a high H+ and a low OH- is an alkaline. In the human body, the pH varies depending on location within the body, for instance, urine pH is 6.0, saliva pH is 6.8, and tears pH is 7.2, etc. The figure below shows the variant pH range in the gastrointestinal tract.

pH of the gastrointestinal tract

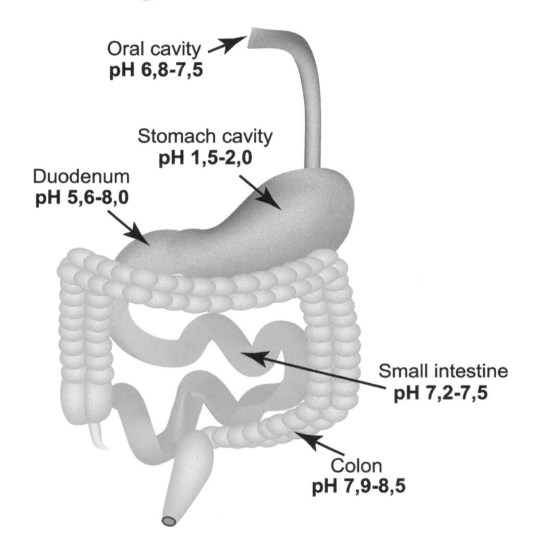

Oral cavity
pH 6,8-7,5

Stomach cavity
pH 1,5-2,0

Duodenum
pH 5,6-8,0

Small intestine
pH 7,2-7,5

Colon
pH 7,9-8,5

Maintaining the Balance in the pH Buffering System

As stated, the pH of the body may be different but the variations are limited and quite specific and remain relatively constant in that area. This balance or homeostasis is maintained by what is called the **buffering system.** When an acid or base are taken into the body the buffering system reacts by trying to balance the orally taken acid or base with a weak acid or base to try and maintain proper pH balance and bring it back to the body's normal pH. These buffers are found in the body's fluids. There are several buffer systems in the body but the most important one is the **carbonic acid-bicarbonate buffer system.** Buffering reaction occurs when one concentration either increases while the other decreases. This is why the buffer system is sometimes called the chemical sponges.

Chemical/Electrolyte Balance in the Older Population

With the aging process, there are cells that are degenerating in the body and these cells are aging at different stages throughout the body. The cells of the stomach and intestinal tract, as well as, other organs of the body will eventually go through this senescence process and this may eventually hit the kidneys and the liver. Once senescence hits these organs, they may cause electrolyte abnormalities that may affect the ability to excrete waste and diluted urine. This will affect the acid, base balance and the salt elimination from the body. Hyponatremia and hypernatremia are common electrolyte abnormalities that may develop in the elder adult. Elder adults tend not to drink enough water or eat a balanced diet as they should and this plus the onset of illness, decline in cognitive ability, and the use of medication can all contribute to this unbalance and trigger electrolyte changes and inadequacy in the acid, base, and salt stability in the body. Chemical electrolytes occasionally can fluctuate due to underlying medical factors and conditions as well.

Symptoms of Electrolyte Imbalance

Electrolyte imbalance can manifest as:

> - **Slow heart rate**
> - **Weakness and exhaustion**
> - **Dry mouth with excessive thirst**
> - **Dizziness**
> - **Reduced coordination and orientation**
> - **Palpitations**
> - **Hypotension (low blood pressure)**
> - **Nausea and possible regurgitation/vomiting**
> - **Muscle spasm and/ or cramps**
> - **Irritableness and change in temperament**

It is important to be aware of this potential electrolyte imbalance in the elder adult and take steps to prevent this disorder. If any of these signs present themselves or you are experiencing some of the above symptoms it is vital to call your doctor and/or family member for advice. Medication can present with untoward side effects that may mimic similar symptoms. Hormone fluctuations, gastric irrationality, and liver or kidney diseases must be treated. There are some electrolyte drinks such as Propel water, Powerade, Bodyarmor, Emergen-c, Gatorade, Pedialyte, and many more. These electrolyte enhanced drinks can be useful as sports drinks to help replenish water and electrolytes and increase energy that is lost. It can also be useful for the elder population in maintaining electrolyte balance. Electrolyte drinks may contain vitamins, potassium, sodium, magnesium, and calcium and will help combat dehydration, prevent muscle cramps, and increase vitality hopefully preventing more complications.

ELECTROLYTES

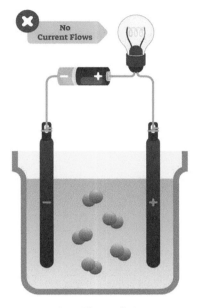

Nonelectrolyte

Ethanol

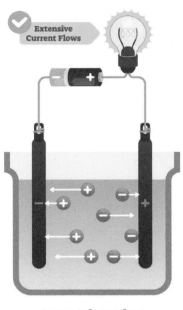

Strong Electrolyte

Sodium Chloride

| No Current Flows |
| Extensive Current Flows |

An Electrolyte is a Substance that will Conduct Electricity when Dissolved in Water or When Molten

All Salts and some Polar Covalent Compounds are Electrolytes

EXAMPLE

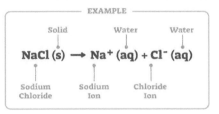

$$NaCl\ (s) \longrightarrow Na^+\ (aq) + Cl^-\ (aq)$$

Solid → Water, Water

Sodium Chloride | Sodium Ion | Chloride Ion

THE MAIN ELECTROLYTES IN BODY FLUID

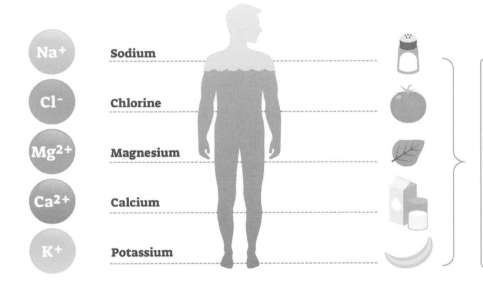

Na^+ Sodium

Cl^- Chlorine

Mg^{2+} Magnesium

Ca^{2+} Calcium

K^+ Potassium

Balance Fluids in Your Body

Maintain Your Blood's Proper pH

Carry Electrical Signals from Nerves to Muscles

Chapter 3

Musculoskeletal System

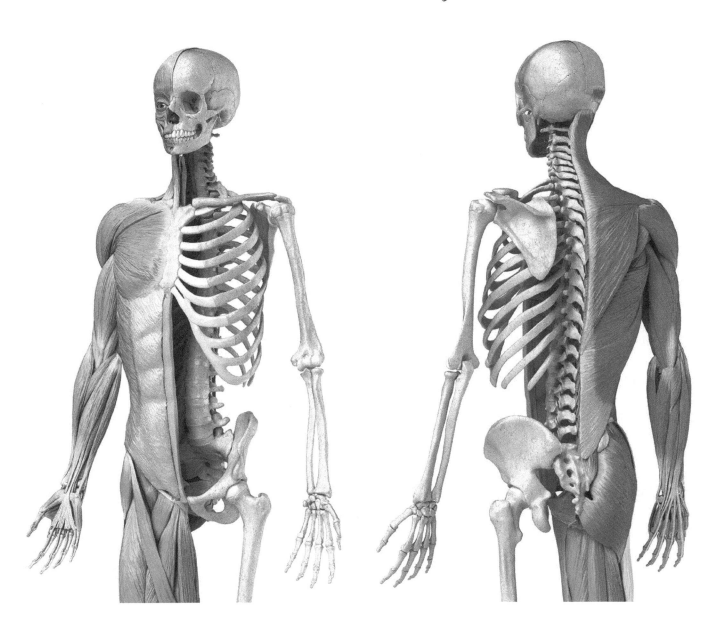

Contents in Chapter 3

Musculoskeletal System

When manufactures build a car they first must build the frame or structure of the car. This structure must have a means of movement so at the ends there are hinges or pivot points that are fashioned with levers, joints and leverages, coils, pulleys, tensions, and many other implements and machinational technologies that are used like wheels to make it mobile. The mechanical apparatus of an engine must be installed with piston ignition system mounted into the frame to give it the potential of power for movement and this must be installed and connected to the turning apparatus with a turn system that controls and moves the wheels on the ground. Switches must be installed to allow internal control of the engine and so much more has to be mounted but after all this structure on this framework it is still just a heap of metal. Energy has to be found and given to this engine for it to achieve its full potential: the ability to move under its own power. The power for this potential movement comes from the energized battery, the gasoline, diesel or an electricity charged system which will ignite the fuel to move the pistons and eventually to allow this heap of metal to move and become what it was built to be: an automobile.

The human skeletal system

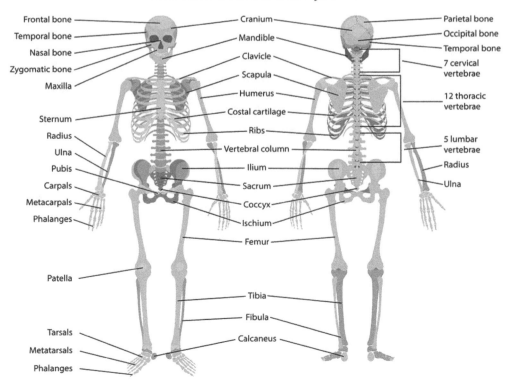

Bones and Their Function

The body is the same way, though much more imaginative. There are 206 bones in the human body that make up the skeletal system. The skeletal system is the framework of the body that has ligaments and cartilages as hinges and pivot points to allow bending with the potential of movement. To understand how these bones can eventually move with the help of the muscles system or engine you need to learn the parts of the bones, the hinges and the pivot points which the muscles are going to eventually be attached. In the human body these 206 bones support the body, protect its organs, store and supply the body with needed lipids and calcium, and produce blood cells needed for the body. These bones are in different shapes and forms or structures, for instance, the bones of the chest are shaped as a cage to house and protect the lungs and heart. This chest cage is called the thorax area or ribs and is able to expand and relax on inhalation and exhalation as well as go up and down. The bones of the cranium or skull are flat and are shaped as a vault or cavity and these flat bones cover and protect the brain and its contents from harm. For movement, bones are placed in close proximity to each other to come together as a pivot area called a joint or **articulation.** Medical professionals use bony landmarks to locate vital organs such as the heart and lungs, blood vessels and nerves around or close to the bony structures. These bony landmark locations are called **"The Anatomic Position."**

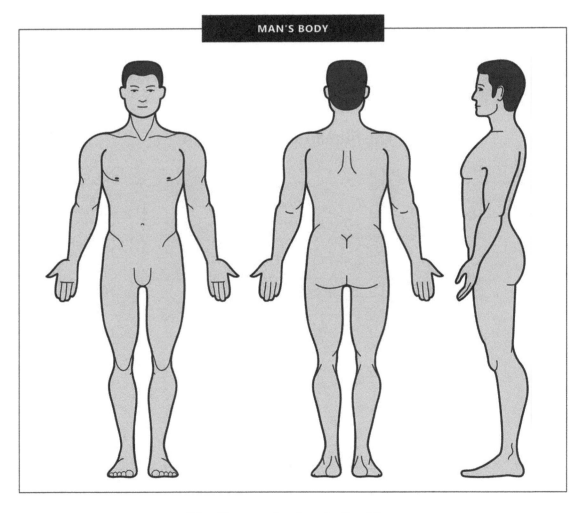

MAN'S BODY

The Human Anatomic Position

Anatomic Position

The anatomic position are reference points that serves as a guide for medical professionals to use in locating specific areas on the human body for medical view and evaluation and in describing specific parts of the human anatomy. In this anatomic position, the subject stands erect facing the observer with the head level and the eyes facing forward. The feet are flat on the floor and directed forward, and the upper limbs are at the side with palms side facing forward.

Bone Function

1. **Support** – It provides support and protection for the organs, soft tissues, and attachments such as the ligaments and tendons for the skeletal muscles.
2. **Protection** – The skeleton protects the most important internal organs from injury.
3. **Assistance in movement** – The skeletal muscles attach to various bones; when the muscles contract, they pull on the bones to produce movement.
4. **Mineral Storage** – The bones store several minerals, especially calcium and phosphorus of which contributes to the bone's strength.
5. **Blood cell reproduction** – Certain bones called red bone marrow produces red blood cells, white blood cells, and platelets.
6. **Triglyceride storage** – Yellow bone marrow consist mainly of adipose cells which stores triglycerides. This storage of triglycerides is a potential chemical energy reserve.

Bones and its Classification

The hardest tissues in the human body are the teeth and the bones. This hardness is due to the various types of cells, minerals, and **collagen fibers** within its matrix. As stated, bones have various shapes, sizes, and some are even oddly and irregularly shaped but they all serve the body's functions and needs. When classified by shape there are flat bones, long bones, short bones and irregular bones.

Flat bones are generally two thin plates of compact bones fitted together with a layer of underlying spongy central region of bone which is called the **diploe.** They afford protection at the areas of attachment for the flat bones. Flat bones include cranial bones (protects the brain), sternum and rib bones (protect the organs of the chest), bones of the pelvis, and the scapulae.

Long bones have a greater length than width and are slightly curved for strength. They have a shaft called **diaphysis** and two ends called **epiphysis.** Long bones are meant to absorb weight so the stress is evenly distributed. Bones of the thigh, legs, toes, arms forearms, and fingers are examples of long bones.

Short bones are block or cube-shaped and nearly equal in width and length. It is spongy in texture and compact at the surface. Examples of a short bone are the wrist and ankle bones.

Irregular bone shapes vary, such as, the vertebrae column which has wings or buttresses for attachments of muscles, tendons, and ligaments. Certain facial bones are also irregular in shape. There are other irregular bones in the body, such as, the **sutural bone** and **Wormian bones** found in the suture line of the cranium (skull), the **sesamoid bones** found in the foot, thumb, patella, and pisiform of the knee.

Long Bone Structure

The structure of the long bone of the upper leg is the shaft or diaphysis and at the two ends of the shaft are the epiphyses. The diaphysis is hollow called the **medullary cavity** but the outer wall is composed of compact bones that are very dense and hard. The medullary cavity interior is composed of **marrow** and is where the red blood cells develop. The long bone or diaphysis is covered with a connected tissue called the periosteum. Blood vessels are in the center of the marrow and this is where **osteoblast** cells are developed and form compact bones that continue to the outer surface but not in the interior of the bone. A typical long bone consists of the following:

- **Diaphysis** – Is the bone's shaft or body of the bone and is a long cylindrical main portion of the bone structure.
- **Bone marrow** – Within the diaphysis called the medullary cavity is where there is bone marrow. The bone marrow is red in children and yellow in adults.
- **Epiphyses** – Are the proximal and distal ends of the bone.
- **Trabecular (spongy)** – Within the epiphyses there is the trabecular or spongy bone that contains red bone marrow.
- **Articular cartilage** – Is a thin layer of cartilage covering the epiphyses where the bone forms an articulation (joint) with another bone.
- **Periosteum** – Is the external surface of the bones.

Once the structure of the bone is formed the osteoblast or bone forming cells continue to form throughout the life of the person and it is the **osteoclast** or bone destroying cells that dissolves the bone and provides the body with calcium and phosphate. These minerals are necessary for cell metabolism and heart function. Normally there is a balance between osteoblast and osteoclast but as we age this balance may alter or change and less osteoblast will form with more osteoclast or bone breakdown of cells being produced with a greater loss of calcium. This happens in older adults and this loss of calcium from the bone's weakness the compactness of the bones causing the bones to be brittle which can develop into a complex condition called **osteopenia** which may cause **osteoporosis.** Diet changes and supplements may be recommended to prevent, stop, or improve this condition: more on this in a later chapter.

Joints and Articulations

Although bones are separate units, they are held together and connected to each other by flexible joints. These joints allow the movement of that particular part of the body. The study of the joints is called **arthrology.** Joints are junctions that allow specific types of movements between two or more bones. A joint is also called an **articulation or arthrosis** and is a point of contact between other bones, between bone and **cartilage,** or between bones and teeth. When we use the word **articulate,** we mean that the bones form a joint. A joint is bound by ligaments. Ligaments are tissues that cross over the joints and muscles, thereby connecting bone to bone. Joints:

1. Allows movement of the body
2. Cartilage is connective tissue to the bone – Articular cartilage reduces the friction of the bone and acts as a shock absorber.

Types of Joints

Although there are a number of different forms of joints in the human body, they can be easily classified by their movement or lack of movement. These include immovable, slightly movable, freely movable, ball-and-socket, and hinge joints. We will describe just five of these joints as follows:

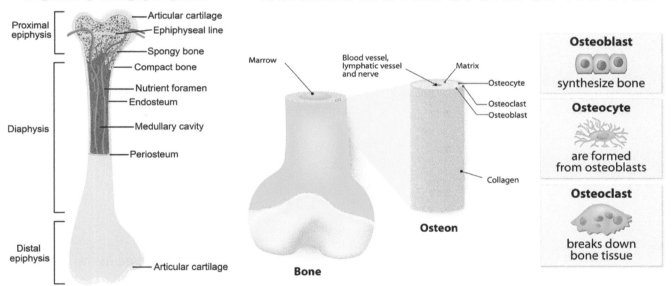

> **Immovable joint or synarthroses joint** is formed by interlocking edges and are found between the bones such as the suture lines in the skull.
> **Slightly movable joint or amphiarthroses joint** – are joints formed by adjacent vertebrae containing intervertebral disc forms of cartilage. Vertebral column.
> **Ball-and-socket or diarthroses** – Allows movement in three planes at one time (3-degree joint movement at one time). Example: Shoulder and hip
> **Hinge joint or diarthroses** – Allows movement in one plane (1-degree of freedom). Example: Elbow and knee
> **Gliding joint or diarthroses** – Allows movement in three planes (3-degree of freedom). Example: Wrist and feet

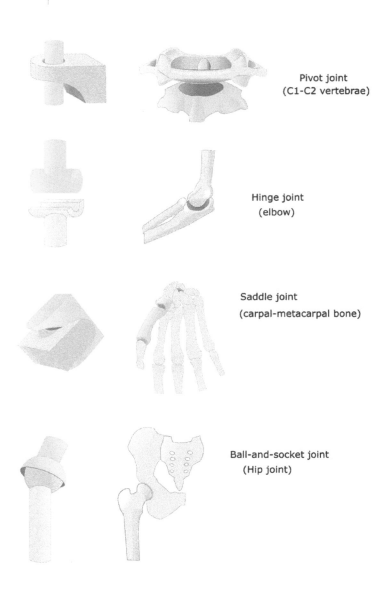

Pivot joint
(C1-C2 vertebrae)

Hinge joint
(elbow)

Saddle joint
(carpal-metacarpal bone)

Ball-and-socket joint
(Hip joint)

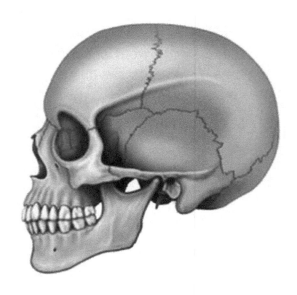

Sutural/Wormian joints in the cranium

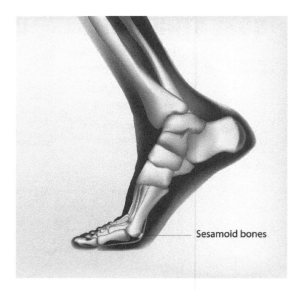

Sesamoid bones

Sesamoid bones in the foot

Skeletal Movement – Joints and Muscles

It is the muscles that enable the skeletal body to move via the joint system. The muscle's tendon is attached to the bones and interfaces at cross angles to the joints. The attachment or interfaces closest to the center of the body is the **proximal attachment (PA)** and is also called the muscle **origin (O).** It is the muscle fibers that are directly affixed to the bone. The muscle attachment that interfaces away from the center of the body is the **distal attachment (DA).** It is also called the **insertion (I).** Muscle tendons extend, usually across one or more joints and when the muscle contracts they pull the bone and movement is achieved.

How Aging Affects the Joints

Age has no exceptions as to gender or how one maintains their health throughout the years. Time always wins out. As one ages, the body cells start to change and this goes for the cells of the bones and the joints in the human body. As one becomes older, the ligaments that connect bone to bone become stiffer and more brittle and the tendons grow older and become less flexible prone to fraying, tearing, stiffening, and breaking causing pain and injury to the individual. It will cause **ROM or range of motion** changes and this will affect the way you walk, bend, stand, reach and/or rise-up from a chair. Changes in bones will also have an effect on joint mobility because it directly involves the articular cartilage that is undergoing reduction in density, loss of synovial fluid, flexibility, overall effectiveness, and loss in tissue homeostasis with the resulting loss of smooth coordinated motor skills. This change is not uniform throughout the body and this reduction change will affect different joints at different times and/or in different degrees of stiffness, discomfort, and restriction. Those that have a more active lifestyle will experience this later in life then the more sedentary person. Eventually, all will be affected and some of us will start to lose joint lubricating fluid. Without this synovial lubrication fluid, the joints will eventually start to rub together against the other bones causing an inflammatory condition called **osteoarthritis.**

The Muscular System

Providing the framework of bones, joints, ligaments, and leverages to this structure still does not make the structure move. It needs an engine or muscle action attachments to the bones: a fixed end called the origin and a movable area called the insertion to fit that profile. As stated, the origin of a tendon is normally close to the body's midline and the insertion of tendon is usually distant from the body's midline with some origins and insertions having multiple attachment areas of function. The tendons are what is attached to the bones and these tendons vary in lengths and strengths depending on their use, location, needs, and function. No one muscle action moves a body part. It takes two or more muscles acting together to move a body part, one action for contraction or to bring the body part closer to the body and one action for extension returning the body part away from the body. A good example of this would be the muscles of the arm (elbows) and legs (knees) that are hinge joints. The biceps muscle flexes the forearm bringing the hand closer to the face and the triceps muscle extends or stretches allowing contraction to work. When the contraction is completed, the triceps muscle contracts returning the forearm back to its original position bringing the hand away from the face.

Characteristics, Structure, and Function of the Muscular System

There are four basic characteristics of muscle tissue, the ability to receive stimuli or **excitability,** the ability to shorten and thicken as in **contractility,** the ability of the muscle to stretch to continue the contract and range of resting lengths **extensibility,** and the ability of the muscle to rebound towards the original length **elasticity.** This allows motion for the body as well as the production of heat to maintain body temperature. The muscle cells itself are surrounded by a connective tissue fiber called **endomysium** (one muscle cell). The **muscle bundle,** also called the motor unit, (two or more muscle cells), and this is surrounded by a sheath of connective tissue called the **perimysium.** The entire muscle group, such as the bicep muscle, is surrounded by a sheath of connective fibrous tissue (two or more muscle bundles/motor units) called the **epimysium.** The epimysium is the extension of **deep fascia** (a sheet of fibrous connective tissue) that divides the muscles into bundles of fibers called **fascicules.** All of this just for the soul function to;

1) **Produce movement** – to allow muscle and tendons to move the skeletal bones,
2) **Maintain posture and body position** – to maintain all movement of the body,
3) **Support the tissue** – to shield and protect abdominal walls and other organs in the body,
4) **Guard entrances and exits** – to allow openings in the digestive and urinary tracts,
5) **Maintain body temperature** – when muscles contract, energy is required and when used this energy produces heat.

Types of Muscle Fibers/Tissues

There are approximately 656 to 700 muscles in the human body. Out of this there are three types of muscle fibers: **cardiac muscle fiber, skeletal muscle fiber, and smooth muscle fiber.** The cardiac muscle fibers are the muscle fibers of the heart and is an involuntary muscle, the smooth muscle fibers are the muscles of the intestinal tract and is also an involuntary muscle fiber, and the skeletal muscles fibers which are also called the striated muscles and these are voluntary and involuntary muscle fiber.

Structure of Skeletal Muscle

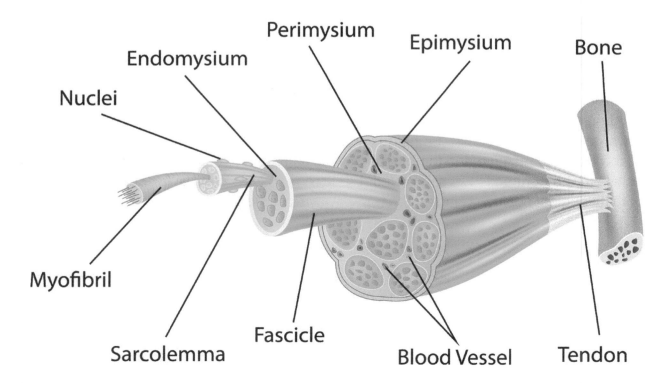

There is so much more to go over in the anatomy and physiology of the muscular system that it would take up much too much time to discuss. What is important in this very brief discussion on the development of the muscular system and what we will concentrate on in this transitory brief is the aging process of the muscular system.

Types of Muscle Tissue

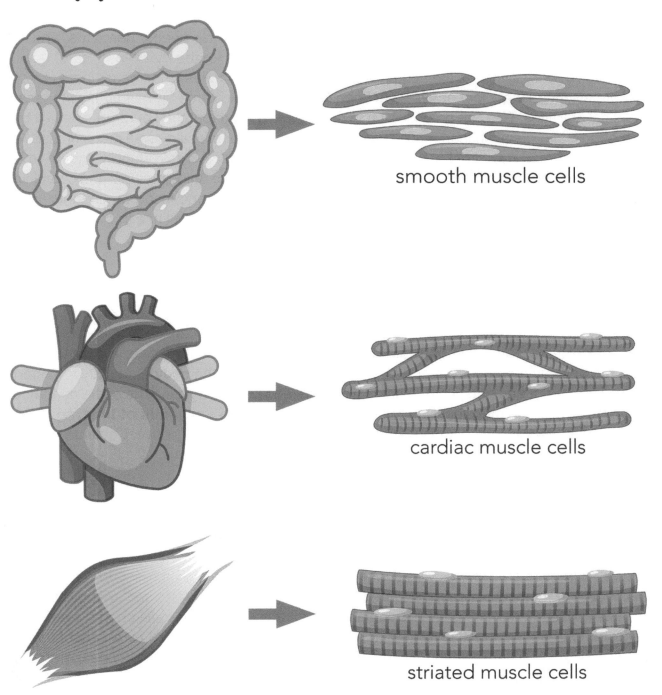

smooth muscle cells

cardiac muscle cells

striated muscle cells

Aging of the Muscle Tissues

There is no absolute age as to when the skeletal muscle strength decreases or becomes less flexible and starts to lose their lean strength and mass. There are some scientists that think that this can start early around the age of 30 to 50 years depending on the individual's physical activities. There is actual evidence that at age 50 there is significant loss of lean muscle strength and mass. This percentage is across the board for both genders with women losing less overall muscle mass. Muscle loss due to age is called **sarcopenia** (sarco=muscle and penia=waste) and this can change an individual's quality of life. The loss of mitochondria and the decrease in the muscle proteins will have an effect on muscle mass, strength, and tone. Not only will it have an effect on you in a physiological way but in a social and personal way. It has an overall effect on the health and wellness of the person in regards to the needs, demands, and the dependence in utilizing medical and social services resources for the maintenances of quality of life needs of daily living. As the senior citizen population continues to increase, there is more and more evidence that older adults have been keeping pace in some form or other with regard to physical activities. This can be observed in most gyms throughout the country. It is a fact that active people can maintain lean muscle strength longer and lose less muscle mass at a slower rate than the normal stay at home person so becoming a more active individual is a good way of slowing down sarcopenia. This alone will help in slowing down the aging process and combining this with the reduction in stress and learning Yoga or meditation and incorporating this with a healthy diet will increase the chance tenfold of maintaining your overall health overtime.

Sports and the Aging Muscles

There is a time when professional athletes must face the fact that it is time to call it a well-earned and well performed career. Many athletes try to pass their physical time limit to achieve more than their body's ability to give. This is because the mind says "yes I can" and the body says "no I cannot extent it anymore." Your body always wants to remain physically active, in this there is no doubt, but being in a competitive and challenging mode behind the body's capacity to perform is just a fail's arrant and puts a strain on all biological and psychological parts of the mind/body capability, not just the muscles. Nobody wins when it comes to the **sands of time**. Aging is a normal human journey but it does not mean that you should remain inactive. Continue physical activities and enjoy the fruits of this action for as long as you can.

How this aging process progresses is the real story. Lean body muscle mass tissue loss is a normal and expected part of the aging process but this is not just the only loss. According to scientific research (The Scientist Daily Newsletter – TSDN), muscle aging is due to the decrease in muscle stem cells, mitochondrial dysfunction, a decline in proteins quality and turnover, and hormonal deregulation. This is evident when it comes to muscle strength and endurance and is secondary to the diminished muscle mass and its ability in catabolism and anabolism or the synthesis and break-down of protein. Decrease in endurance can be associated with a reduction in mitochondria and its abilities to absorb oxygen from the blood caused by a sedentary and inactive life style which is the main reason for the loss of strength but there is hope regardless of age. The skeletal muscles of the human body are amazing and very impressive when it comes to exercise. It has what TSDN calls **"Plasticity"** or the quality of being easily shaped and molded:

that is the muscular system. Age should not hold you up if you want to exercise. Although it is nice to start at an earlier age, exercise has no age limit. By exercising, you can increase your strength and mass as well as slow down sarcopenia **period.** There is an abbreviation you should put to memory **S.A.I.D.,** that is, **Specific Adaptions to Imposed Demands** which basically means that your body muscles has the ability to adapt to any stresses, difficulties, or activities you put upon it, such as, a safe and appropriate amount of exercise in a well-planned program or training endeavor with demands that are put upon the skeletal muscles system. You can gain mass and strength through this training in an appropriate period of time. You can start now or at any age just like that of any young person and achieve the same results that a younger person can achieve; this includes aerobic endurance exercises. This activity does not have to be heavy or hard work, it just has to be above your normal energy expenditures of daily living. This added activity can be as simple as a walk around the block or instead of using the elevator walking up and down the steps. It is strongly suggested that one should join a gym or aerobics class, though exercising at home will work. You just have to move about more, garden or use the stairs as exercise. There is no such thing as "I don't have the time" or "I don't have the money." Just do it!

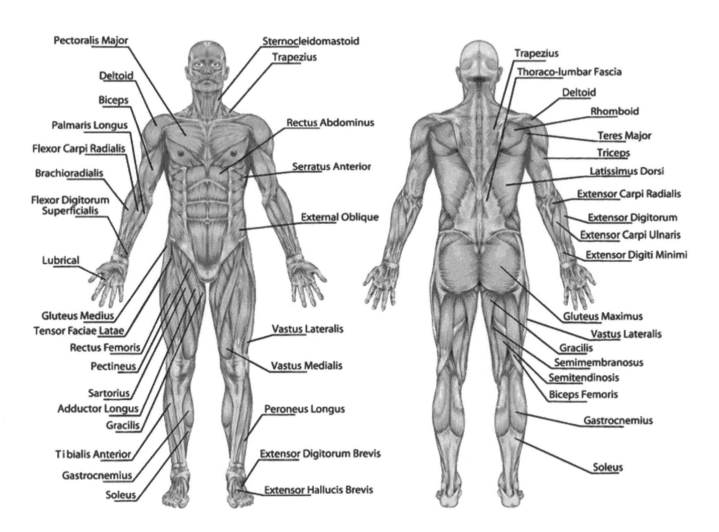

Chapter 4

The Nervous System:
Structure, Function, and Organization

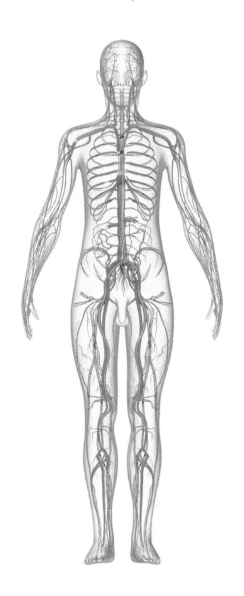

Contents in Chapter 4

The Nervous System: Structure, Function, and Organization

A very basic introduction into the nervous system is essential in learning of the neurophysiology, medical, and cognitive aspects of the nerves and the brain as we age. This neuropath is responsible for the complex relationship between the internal human body environment and its connection to the external environment. This connection, in a broad sense, involves two organ systems which coordinates together to give us information about our location in space and time, condition, and brief response to our surroundings. These two organ systems are the **nervous system** and the **endocrine system.** The nervous system gives us a swift but a brief response to a stimulus whereas the endocrine system gives us a much more controlled and slower response method but one that is a longer lasting response command. The body's internal environment and the external environment are linked to these two systems by our senses of touch, smell, sight, hearing, taste, feeling, and other mental awareness that are unclassified responses of which we instinctively respond to. Some of these responses are our physical or voluntary responses and others are our body's automatic internal ability of responses.

Division of the Nervous System

There are two separate divisions of the nervous system: the **central nervous system (CNS)** and the **peripheral nervous system (PNS).** The brain is the overall control center and the spinal cord is the transport system of the human body's central nervous center. All communication from the central nervous system for the body comes through the PNS which includes all neural tissue outside the CNS. There are two divisions of the CNS: the **afferent division** which brings sensory information to the CNS and **efferent division** which carries motor commands to various areas of the body like the muscles and glands. The efferent division is divided into two areas; the **somatic nervous system (SNS)** that provides voluntary control of the muscles and the **autonomic nervous system (ANS)** which is the involuntary movement of the cardiac, intestinal, stomach, and other autonomic muscle activities.

Organization of the Neural Tissues

The neural tissues also called the nervous system is all the nerves in the human body of which there are two basic components of cells: the two basic units are the **neurons** and

neuroglia. Neurons communicate with one another and with the cells, the **neuroglia** regulates the environment around the neurons (homeostasis) that forms the **myelin sheath** providing support and a framework for the neural tissues in the form of phagocyte or bacteria protectors which in general protect the neuron. The neurons have three functional groups:

1. **Sensory neuron** which is part of the afferent unit that convey or impute information from the external and internal environment
2. **Motor neuron** which is part of the efferent unit that controls and carries instructions from the CNS to the muscles and glands, maintains homeostasis, mental activity, and other tissues and organs systems.
3. **Interneurons** are located entirely in the brain and the spinal cord and they interconnect or integrate the complex information from neurons also analyzing imputes and outputs received by the brain.

There are many shapes, sizes, and purposes of neurons, such as, the **multipolar, the unipolar, and the bipolar neuron** but they all have the same function, to conduct and transmit messages or information. Some examples of the types and shapes of neurons:

TYPES OF NEURONS

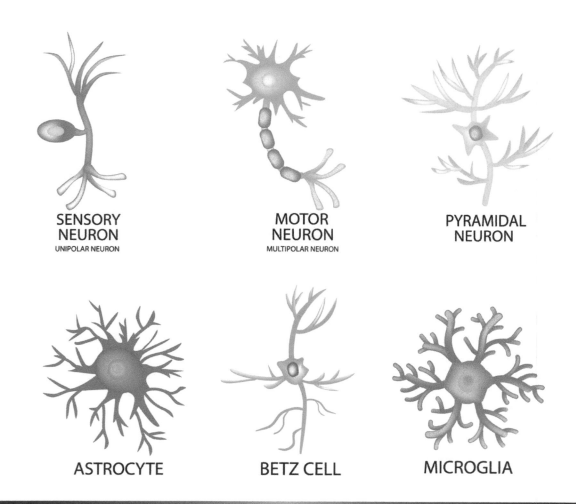

SENSORY
NEURON
UNIPOLAR NEURON

MOTOR
NEURON
MULTIPOLAR NEURON

PYRAMIDAL
NEURON

ASTROCYTE

BETZ CELL

MICROGLIA

The **neuroglia or glial** cells are forms of connective tissue cells that provide support for the neurons. There are ten times as many glial cells then there are neurons in the nervous system. These glial cells are in the CNS and the PNS but the CNS has the greatest diversity of glial cells. There are four types of glial cells and it is important to understand these types because it has a direct influence on the aging process:

1) **Astrocytes** – Secretes chemicals vital to the maintenances of the blood-brain barrier and performs repairs to damaged neural tissue. It isolates the CNS circulation from the general circulation.
2) **Oligodendrocytes** – This is a protective cytoplasmic barrier that is wrapped around the axon called the **myelin sheath** and there are many oligodendrocytes coating the entire axon. The myelin sheath improves the speed and impulse conduction along the line of the axon. There are gaps or spaces in between the myelin sheath that are called the **nodes of ranvier.**
3) **Microglia** – Are the phagocytes cells that migrated across the capillary walls. These white blood cells protect the axons and are similar to the white blood cells of the circulatory system.
4) **Ependymal cells** – These are cells that line the central canal of the spinal cord and the chambers or ventricles of the brain.

Schwann cells are the most important glial cells in the peripheral nervous system (PNS) and they cover every axon outside of the CNS. A Schwann cell may also surround unmyelinated axons; more on this later.

NEURONS AND NEUROGLIAL CELLS

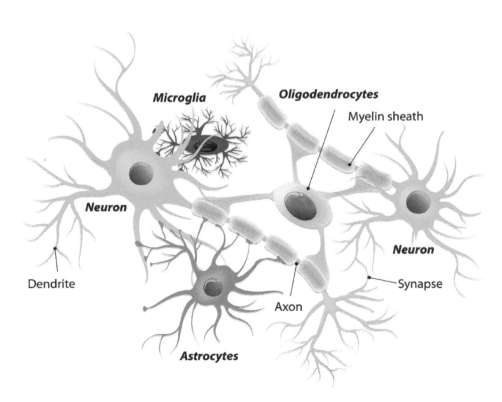

Neuron Structure

There are three distinct portions of the neuron: cell body, dendrites, and axon. The **cell body** is also called the **soma** of which contain several of the organelles of the cell and they are surrounded by **cytoplasm.** These cell body's function to protect and control all cell activities. Organelles are tiny organs within the cell with each organelle having a specific purpose. Out of these organelles, the **nucleus** is the most important because it contains the DNA which regulates all cell function. Within the nucleus is where the **nucleolus** resides and the nucleolus is where the RNA is located. This is the place where the production code is sent for protein synthesis formation. Other organelles are the **mitochondria, Golgi body's, lysosomes,** and the **Nissl body.** In the Nissl body is an accumulation of organelles known as the **rough endoplasmic reticulum** or **(RER)** and is where the proteins are synthesis.

Dendrites are thick cytoplasmic branches with many extensions that contain **chromatophilic** substances, mitochondria, and other organelles for the conduction of impulse toward a cell body. The **axon** is a long, thin, singular, and highly specialized body that has cytoplasmic extension called **axoplasm** and the membrane is called **axolemma** or **neurilemma** also spelled **neurolemma.** The dendrites receive impulses and conducts these impulses away from the cell body to other neuron tissues. Dendrites contain mitochondria and **neurofibrils** but no chromatophilic substances which basically means, it does not carry on protein synthesis. The dendrite's surface is covered with thousands of spines that form junctions with other neurons. At the distal end of the axon junction, there are thousands of microscopic branches called **axon terminals** that have large dotted studs called **synaptic knob nerve cells** that release a chemical called **neurotransmitters.** These neuron transmitters conduct impulses from the neuron to the muscle, gland or other neurons or where ever the pulse is needed in the body. A neurotransmitter is an **endogenous** chemical (a chemical that originates within an organism) that allows transmission signals across a chemical **synapse.** There are over 200 substances that contribute to synaptic transmission: acetylcholine (ACh), Dopamine, epinephrine, norepinephrine, serotonin, glycine, Gamma-aminobutyric acid (GABA), and adenosine just to mention the more common ones.

The Myelin Sheath and Neurolemma

The myelin sheath of the axon of the peripheral nervous system are flattened cells called the neurolemmo-cytes or **Schwann glial cells** which are located along the line of the axons. It encircles and overlaps the axon and winds around it many times and after about 20-30 raps the neurolemmo-cytes membrane becomes the myelin sheath with the outer layer becoming the neurolemma (myelin sheath of Schwann). This neurolemma is found in the PNS and its function is to transmit information to the glands and muscles or other sensory organs like the skin as well as regenerating injured axons. There are gaps of unmyelinated areas called **neurofibral nodes (nodes of Ranvier)** and they start to form late in fetal development and increase from birth to maturity. The central nervous system also has a myelin sheath but it is formed by the oligodendrocytes glial cells and not the Schwann cells. It is important to understand that nerves consist of several bundles of axons known as **fascicle** and each fascicle is surrounded by a sheath called **perineurium.** An **epineurium** fibrous tissue surrounds the nerve and binds them to other fascicles. The neuron cell bodies are grouped together in a mass called a **ganglion** (plural for ganglia) and many exist outside the spinal cord extending the axons to other parts of the body. When the nervous system is activated to respond to a stimulus it is received in the information gathering area celled the **reception** point to be processed. Once it is gathered in the reception area from the external environment and processed, the next step is the **transmission** area where the information is delivered by sensory neuron to the CNS.

MYELIN SHEATH FORMATION STAGES

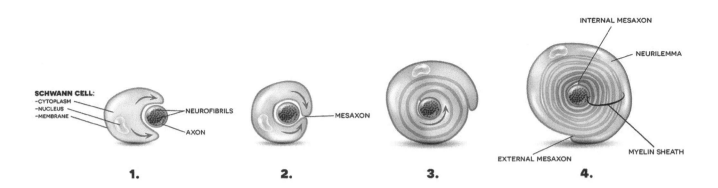

Integration is the third step and it is here that an appropriate response is determined. The final step is the **response step** and in this area a nerve impulse is dispatched to the motor neuron for motor action or stimulus which is the muscles and/or glands the main **effectors** of the body. This is the nervous systems primary nerve physiology.

Nerve Activation and Impulse

We have talked about how the nervous system is stimulated by way of the receptors, transmission, integration, and the response to activate the effectors but how does this all come about. Well, when the nerves are activated, organized neural circuits of the neuron come close to the dendrite of the next neuron along the line of the circuit and this closeness is called the **synapse** (meaning to bring it together). The simplest of these neural circuit stimulations to the effect are the **reflex arc** which begins at the receptor and ends at an effector such as the knee-jerk reflex or the withdrawal reflex which do not involve the brain to activate the response but are automatic responses without conscious thought. There are many receptors in the body and among them are the sense of smell, sight, touch, taste as well as the ones in the skin that determine the temperature. This response is transmitted to the CNS via the sensory neuron through an electrochemical event from an ion in the nerve cell. There are two specific routes in the nerve pathway, the spinal nerve connection and the cranial nerve path connection: more on this later. It is important to understand that when the cell membrane in the muscle and nerve cells are at rest this is called the **resting potential.** There is a considerable difference in the amount and concentration of ions inside and outside these cell plasma membranes so there is no transmission of an impulse. This difference is the result of the distribution of the potassium (K+) ions and the sodium (Na+) ions and their location outside or inside of the cell membrane. In the resting neuron, the K+ concentration is greater in the inside (negatively charged) than the outside of the membrane (positively charged). Even when the nerve cell is not conducting an impulse it is still transporting K+ ions across the membrane and Na+ also; this is called the **sodium-potassium pump** and this action still requires energy or ATP. In the active potential there is more potassium outside the cell membrane and a higher concentration of sodium inside the cell. A nerve impulse is generated called the **action potential** phase and it is when an electrical, chemical, and/or mechanical stimulus is generated. This is caused when there is an alteration in the resting potential and an increase in the permeability of the plasma membrane to sodium which depolarizes the resting potentials. Once depolarized, the sodium ion enters into the cell for a fraction of a second then the channels close and a reversal in polarity occurs. This action potential continues to depolarize adjacent areas and so-on-and-so-forth and this is called **wave of depolarization** which is spreading the chain reaction from area to adjacent area. Once the action potential ends the membrane starts to repolarize and the sodium gate closes and the potassium gate opens causing potassium to flow out of the membrane. Once sodium is out of the neuron the resting potential returns to normal this is called **depolarization state,** that is, it cannot transmit another action potential but a very strong stimulus can result in a nerve impulse. This is called the **all-or-none law.**

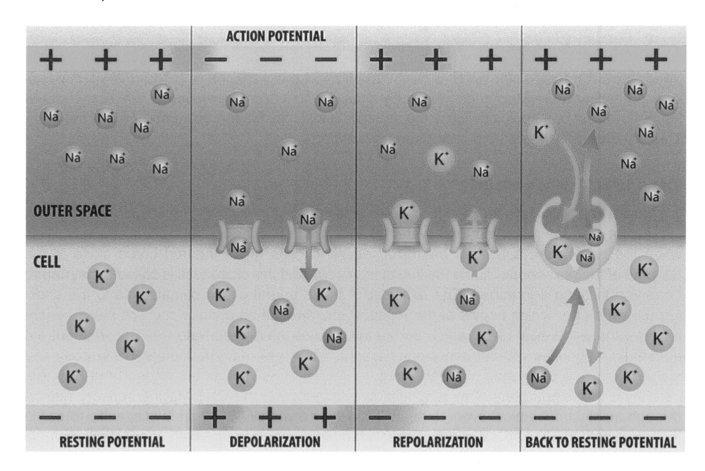

The Synapse

Conduction is not only across the length of the neuron (soma to axon to dendrite) but the impulse conduction is also from neuron to neuron or between neuron to effector muscle or gland. When the conduction is to a muscle it is called a **neuromuscular junction** or **motor end plate** response. The synapse does not actually touch the area it's going to stimulate. There is a space between the synaptic axon vesicles and the effector it's going to stimulate called the **synaptic cleft.** The conducted impulse and the synaptic junction require a neurotransmitter substance to bridge the space or gap to send the message to the receiving effector be it a neuron, muscle, or gland. After the impulse reaches the synaptic knobs at the end of the axons, it triggers a change in the permeability of the neuron that releases neurotransmitting chemicals that diffuses across the synaptic cleft to the effector. This causes a cascade to other dendrites and synapses propagating to other impulses from other neurons.

Anatomy and Organization of the Nervous System

It is the basic function of the nervous system to respond to the action potential that is generated from the individual neurons but the more complex functions occur in the spinal cord and the brain. Neurons and axons are specifically set in the CNS and the PNS in bundles having boundaries that are identified for explicit and defined purposes. To refresh and review: In the PNS the ganglion is neuron cell body's, the nerves represent bundles of axons with spinal nerves connected to the spinal cord and cranial nerves connected to the brain. In the CNS neurons cell body's share a particular function and has an anatomic boundary called the nucleus and in this part of the brain that is covered with a thick gray matter called **neural (meaning nervous cortex)** or just **cortex.** This area is called the brain and it functions as a higher learning center for more complex integration of responses and commands. Tracts connect the bundles of neurons inside the CNS to the spinal cord forming cylindrical columns beginning at the **medulla oblongata** through the **foramen magnum pathways** linking the brain to the rest of the body.

To protect this mass of neural tissue (the brain and spinal cord) is the work of the glial or glia cells within the neural tissue but it also has a series of layers called the **meninges** which house the cerebral spinal fluid and by the special properties within the blood-brain barrier that are semipermeable border that separate the brain circulation with the extracellular fluid circulation. The spinal cord of the adult is white nerve tissue of approximately 18 inches in length that passes through the foramen magnum where it continues with the medulla oblongata to the first or second lumbar vertebrae (T12 to L3). Below that there is a spinal nerve root and meninges. As is in the brain, it is also protected by the glial cells and layers of meninges. The brain is also enclosed within the bony vault of the skull called the cranium and the spinal cord within the bony vertebral column. It is the PNS that informs the CNS of any stimuli received via the axons and dendrites of the motor and sensory neurons from the external environment. The CNS receptors receive the transmission, integrate and interpret the stimuli, then replies to the effector making the stimulus for an appropriate response. Although the outside of the spinal cord is white **(white matter)** the inside is gray **(gray matter)** due to the cell body's-and-neurons.

NEURON ANATOMY

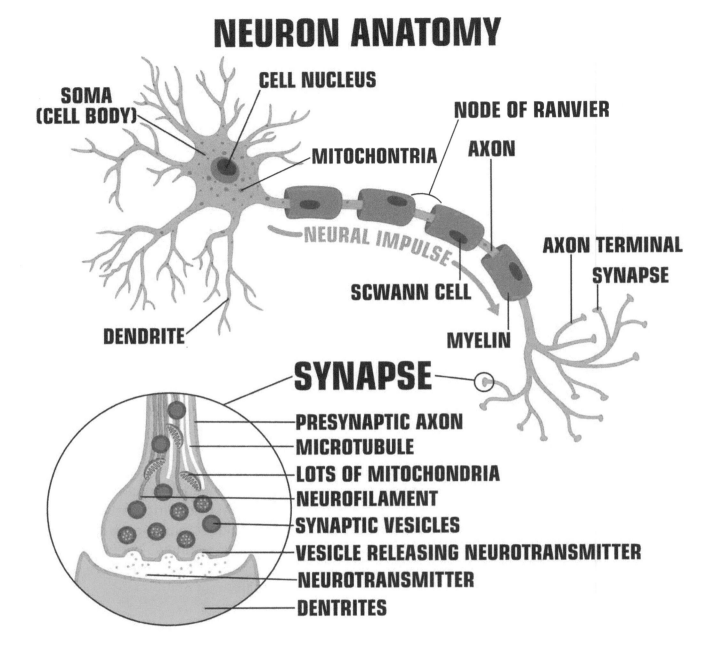

Surrounding and protecting the spinal cord itself there is the same brain tissue the meninges and it is composed of the same three layers of meningeal tissue. These layers are: the dura mater, the arachnoid, and the pia mater.

A. **Dura mater** – The dura mater is attached to and extends from the foramem magnum to the sacrum and coccyx and contains a fibrous connective tissue, many blood vessels, and nerves. The dura mater is the outermost layer of the meninges and does not connect to the vertebral column but is separated by the epidural space and surrounds and supports the dural sinuses. In the brain the dura mater extends inward between the lobes of the brain to form a partition.

B. **Arachnoid mater** – The arachnoid is a loosely fitting thin network of membranes that does not have any blood vessels. The arachnoid traverses from the foramen magnum to the S2 (sacral 2) vertebral region. There is a wide space between the pia mater and the arachnoid called the **subarachnoid space** and it is in this space that contains the **cerebrospinal fluid (CSF).**

C. **Pia mater** – The pia mater is a very thin layer of membrane which contains the most nerves and blood vessels and its envelopes the anterior spinal artery and the median fissure. The medical professionals use it as a surgical landmark.

The spinal cord fluid (CSF) serves as nutrition and to provide gaseous needs for the nerve cells. Along the entire spinal cord there are 31 pairs of projections called **nerve roots** which are the sites of the cell body's and axons of sensory nerves. The ventricle roots on the ventricle side are called the **ventricle nerve roots** which contain the axon for the motor neurons that control muscles and glands, the roots closest to the dorsal side are the dorsal roots and are called **dorsal nerve roots** containing the sensory neurons and injuries to the dorsal roots can lead to anesthesia to the body while injury to the ventricle roots can lead to paralysis of the body. (Remember: sensory=dorsal and ventral=motor roots).

The Spinal Cord

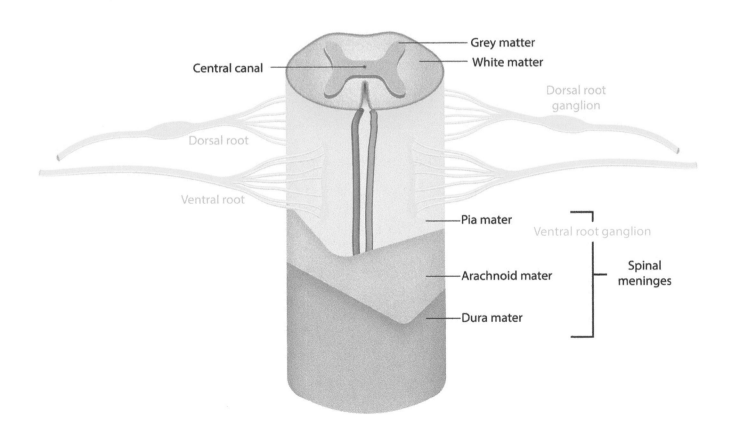

The Brain

The brain weighs approximately 1,300g or 3 pounds in the average adult and is the largest organ in the human body. It is more complex than the spinal cord and is the organizing processing center of the nervous system. It is the site for all consciousness, sensations, and memory in the human condition. The human brain contains almost 98 percent of all the neural tissue which is roughly 38 billion neurons organized into hundreds of **neuronal pools** for various functions. In the individual, there is a variation in the size of the brain due to the difference in gender and the height and weight or the general size of the person but there is no difference in intelligence. The spinal cord is the transportation system of the brain and sends impulses to the brain through 12 pairs of cranial nerves that arise from internal and external environmental senses and other organs. Once the brain interprets the response it sends back to the motor neurons for a response reply through the spinal cord channel. The brain also functions to initiate memory, thoughts, dreams, plans, passions, and coordinated responses to ideas and cognitive intellectual thinking and it is all as a result of brain activity.

Anatomy and Principle Parts of the Brain

The brain has a right and left hemisphere and is protected by the cranial bone and the cranial meninges that completely surrounds the brain of which is continuous with the spinal cord. The spinal cord itself; the outer portion is gray **(gray matter)** and the inner portion is white **(white matter).** The brain and spinal cord have the same protective meninges: dura mater, arachnoid, and the pia mater. The cranial dura mater consists of two layers, the **periosteal layer** that adheres to the cranial bone, a **subdural space** then a thinner smoother **meningeal layer** that envelops the arachnoid mater and corresponds to the spinal dura mater. The lymphatic cerebrospinal fluid CSF further services to protect the central nervous system against injury and this fluid is circulated through the subarachnoid space around the brain, through the ventricles of the brain, and the spinal cord. It has a large capillary system that service to nourish, provide oxygen, exchange gases, and eliminate waste deposited. The brain is extremely sensitive to oxygen consuming 25 percent of the total volume inhaled in the body.

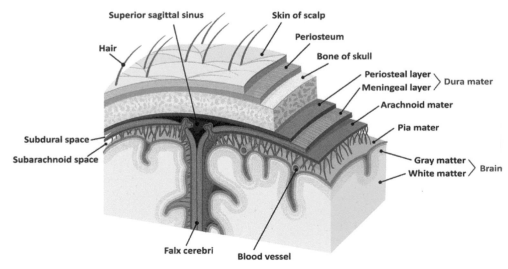

The Cranial Meninges

There are four principle portions of the brain; the brain stem, the diencephalon, the cerebrum, and the cerebellum.

1. **Brain-stem** – is a collection of cerebrum nerve tissue connected to the spinal cord that includes the mesencephalon or midbrain, medulla oblongata, and the pons. The **mesencephalon or midbrain** is associated with vision, hearing, motor control, sleep and wake, arousal (alertness), and temperature regulations. It is next to and joined with the **diencephalon** while posteriorly joined with the pons and cerebellum. The medulla oblongata is the inferior part of the brain and the continuation with the start of the upper spinal cord. It lies superior to the foramem magnum and extends upward to the pons. The medulla connects the ascending and descending tracks for communication with the brain and the spinal cord. Some of these tracts cross from the left pyramid to the right pyramid. As a result of this cross fibers on the left crossing over to the right activate muscles on the right and fibers crossing over to the right activate muscles on the left. This explains why motor areas on one side of the cerebral cortex control muscles of the opposite side of the body. The pons lies directly above the medulla and anterior to the cerebellum and as the word pons means "bridge" it connects the spinal cord to the brain and vis-versa. The pons has paired cranial nerves such as the trigeminal (V) nerve for chewing and sensation of the face and head, the abducens (VI) eyeball movement, etc. to mention a few.

2. **Diencephalon** – this consist of the **thalamus** and the **hypothalamus.** The thalamus serves as the main relay station for sensory impulse except for the sense of smell. It relays vision, taste, hearing, and is the voluntary motor action and arousal area and acts for some interpretation of sensory impulse as pain, temperature touch, and pressure. The hypothalamus deals with external environment originating in the peripheral sense organs such as, sound, taste, smell and somatic responses and uses these senses to control the actions of the autonomic nervous system. It connects with the endocrine system through the pituitary gland with the physiological response to emotional experience.

3. **Cerebrum** – is the largest part of the brain and spreads over the diencephalon. It is about seven-eighths of the total weight of the brain and is concerned with complex memory function. There are two hemispheres connected by nerve fibers called the **corpus callosum.** The cerebrum has many gyri or grooves and a deep groove called a **fissure** and a shallow groove called a **sulcus.** Each hemisphere is divided by four lobes: the frontal lobe is the anterior portion; the parietal lobe is posterior to the frontal lobe; the temporal lobe located below the frontal lobe; and the occipital lobe located at the posterior portion of each hemisphere.

4. **Cerebellum** – is the motor area that regulates activities along the subconscious skeletal motor pathways as the muscles, joints, and tendons by making adjustments in muscle tone, posture, maintaining balance, and programs and fine-tunes voluntary and involuntary movement.

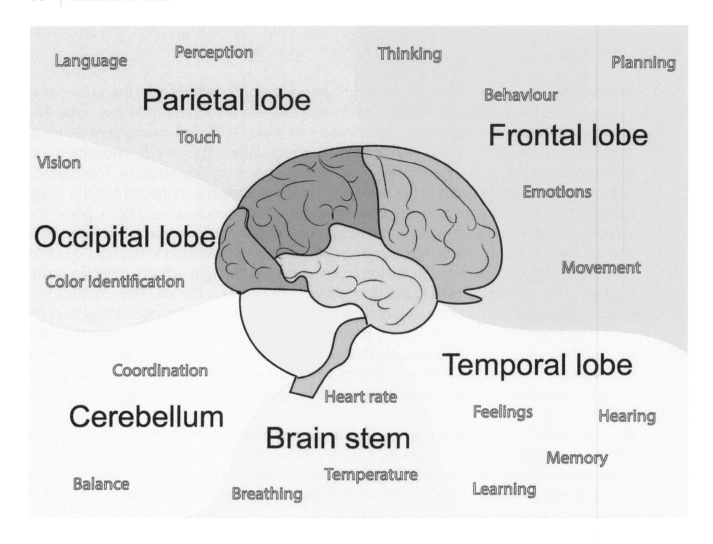

Language Perception Thinking Planning

Parietal lobe

Behaviour

Touch

Frontal lobe

Vision

Emotions

Occipital lobe

Movement

Color identification

Temporal lobe

Coordination

Heart rate

Feelings Hearing

Cerebellum

Brain stem

Memory

Temperature

Balance

Learning

Breathing

The Pineal Gland

This is a gland that is attached to the roof of the midbrain's third ventricle upper surface of the brain and is part of the thalamus. The pineal gland produces **Melatonin.** The production of Melatonin is made during darkness and this Melatonin production is interrupted when light reaches the eyes receptors. Melatonin communicates directly to the brain regulating **circadian rhythm** or the day/night cycles. Melatonin synchronizes the biological clock or circadian rhythm and this rhythm affects the entire body; appetite, energy, mood, and immune system. The pineal gland is believed to regulate secretions of the **gonadotrophic hormone.** This hormone has an effect on reproductive organs, especially of the ovaries and also affects the mating behavior. Other hormones are **adrenoglomerulotropin** that stimulate and secretes **aldosterone** (it controls B/P and at the same time preserving sodium in the body). There are other substances found in the pineal gland, such as, **norepinephrine, serotonin, histamines** to mention just a few. Your brain has other internal clocks in the hypothalamus gland called the **suprachiasmatic nuclei** or **SCN** and this is your body's master clock.

Medial Aspect of the Human Brain

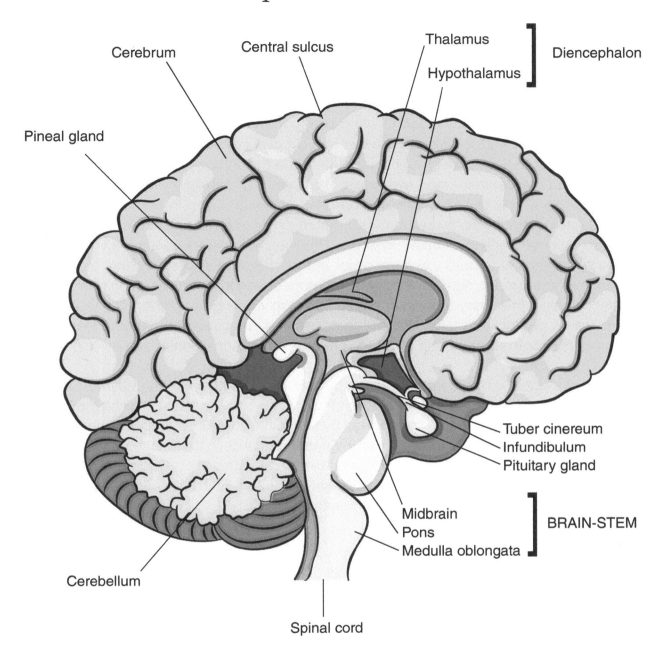

Neurophysiology and the Aging Processes

When we are young the furthest thing from our mind is the idea, fact, concept or dream of one day we will be old. Would it have helped if someone brought this to your attention at an early age? Who knows? It is said that by the age of 30 the brain starts to change, multiple senses in the brain and neuropathways begin to lose their edge and acuteness, which will affect the motor skills slowly reducing its functional awareness. These are all part of the nervous systems aging process. As the aging process continues, our brain and nervous system go through more of this sensory decline and we have difficulty remembering dates, appointments, names, and the abilities of being able to do more than one task at a time. This decline in the aging of the brain and nervous system is not uniform in all aspects of the physiological spectrum or in the cognitive response range. In some individuals body parts, such as, motor or sensory systems will age faster or slower than in other biological parts or with other people in the same age group will have different age response times in their body organs and/or cells. The fact is, there are some that actually become more aware of their environment and are more cognizant in their thinking processes as they grow older. As we go through these natural aging changes certain nerve cells in the brain and spinal cord are lost and circulatory byproducts start to accumulate in the brain and nerve tissue which will contribute to the furtherance of nerve cell breakdown especially around the dendrites and synapses. The myelin sheath Schwann cells of the axon can start to erode and lose their protective barriers and decreasing in function. As we have learned, the nerves are the pathways to messages from the internal and external environment which control voluntary and involuntary systems. This means that the brain and spinal cord that control transport senses in both vis-versa order of the message system pathways as well as what controls all movement, senses, thoughts, memories, and thinking and even normal aging processes, can slow this system down or cause it to stop working altogether. These abnormal factors like waste production that collect at the nerve sites (plaques), tangle, and fatty yellow-brown pigments **(lipofuscin)** can all affect the course of a person's health and their longevity.

When one thinks about it, the central nervous system controls all aspects of every cell in the human body: the skeletal and muscular system, the organs and glands, and all higher learning processes come from the brain and transported by the spinal cords through the central nervous system. It is amazing that the billions of neurons and the glial cells that make up the brain and spinal cord which make multiple connections via axons, dendrites, and synaptic junctions with complex chemical networks can work so flawlessly for years just to become old, slow, and unreliable. Is there a way to slow the aging process down: **YES?**

Chapter 5

Cardiovascular Related Concerns of Aging

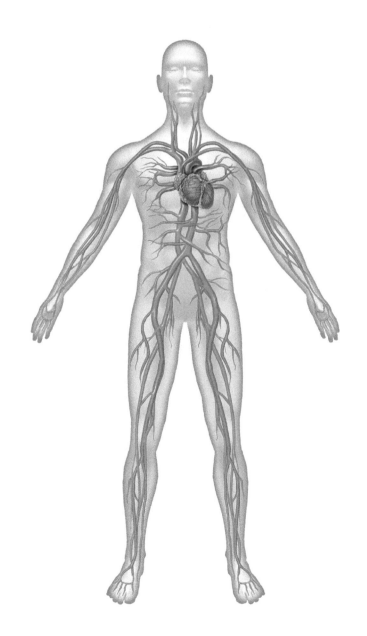

Contents in Chapter 5

Cardiovascular Related Concerns of Aging

Medical and cognitive disorders do not necessarily affect just the older members of the society. As we become older and experience the environmental, sociological, neurological, and economical stressors posed on our mind and body age will overwrought these systems, break them down, and usurp our internal energies, immune system, endocrines system, and cause our muscle strengths to slowly be depleted and/or diminish. It doesn't matter what or how one tries to prevent this from happening: **it is going to happen.** Complications of aging will eventually seep into every cell causing stressors on our lives and risk factors will increase and disorders will develop. As the aging population continues to grow worldwide due to the modernization of our society and advances in health care, the appreciation of preventive health education measures and maintenance improvements, better-quality and understanding of nutritional requirements, improved sanitation knowledge, and with the advancements in our medical care and treatment; there have been and will be more and more adults reaching and passing the age of 70 and at this trend 70 will steadily increase over the years to 80; so-on-and-so-on. The next few chapters will deal with this growing elder population and their medical, neurocognitive, and biological progression as well as the digression effects of aging. Using the congestive heart failure, diabetes mellitus, hypertension, peripheral vascular disease, brittle bones disease syndrome, and dementia mentioned in previous chapters as our guide, we will go into a short didactic overview of the heart and its medical implications in more detail. First, in order to better understand the medical implications of the heart a short preview of the workings of the heart and an outline of the anatomy and physiology of the heart is in order; mainly the structure, function, and purpose.

The Heart: How Does it Work?

Since the heart is one of the major culprits in the **apoptosis** of cell death, it is fitting that we start here. The heart is a strong muscle that pumps blood throughout the body via the cardiovascular system. In a healthy normal adult, the size of the heart is the size of a persons clenched fist. The heart is the engine of the body that keeps the body running. This engine or heart is divided into four chambers, two upper chambers and two lower chambers. The heart is also divided into two sides by a septum and each side has an upper and lower chamber; the upper two chambers are called the right and left atria and the lower two chambers are called the right and left ventricles. The right atrium receives the used poorly oxygenated blood from the body's cells and from the heart for reoxygenation into the circulatory system. Once in the right atrium; this deoxygenated blood is pumped through the tricuspid valves and empties into the right ventricle. From the right ventricle it is pumped through the semilunar valves of the pulmonary system via the pulmonary valves to the pulmonary trunk to the pulmonary arteries to the bronchial tree or lungs. This right atrium to right ventricle through the pulmonary bronchioles into the lungs is called the **pulmonary circuit.** In the lungs the deoxygenated blood and waste products are removed and the blood cells are reoxygenated and sent back to the left atrium then down through the bicuspid valves to the left ventricle. This completes the pulmonary circuit: from the heart to the lungs and back to the heart. The next cycle is the **systemic circuits** where the oxygen rich blood that entered the left ventricle is then pumped through the semilunar aortic valve to the aorta to the rest of the body as well as the left and right coronary arteries. Blood rich oxygen flows to all parts of the body and as the oxygen is used up by the cells, the used or oxygen poor blood or deoxygenated blood returns to the right atrium and the cycle continues.

Cardiac Conduction System

Your heart needs a spark plug to start the engine/heart running and that spark plug is called the **cardiac conduction system.** This conduction system stimulates the muscle of the heart to pulse or pump and this pumping circulates the blood. The spark plug is called the **electrical conduction system** better known as the **cardiac conduction system.** The cardiac muscle cells derive their energy the same way skeletal muscles do, by metabolism, but cardiac muscles require more of the energy so therefore there is more metabolic activity going on in the cardiac cells. The heart has specialized tissues that are connected to the nervous system like a spark plug in a car engine but this one receives nerve stimulation via electrical impulse that transmit signals generated to the node receptors. These nerve node stimulators or nerve impulse receptors contracts the cells of the heart involuntarily (independent of will) and initiates the beating, pumping or pulse that you feel.

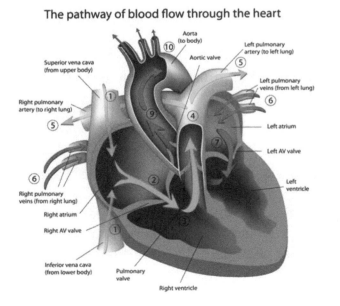

The pathway of blood flow through the heart

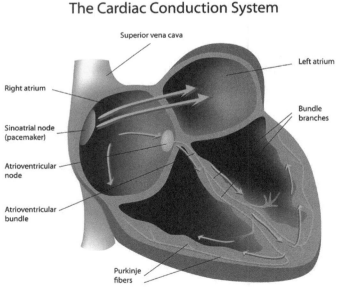

The Cardiac Conduction System

The first component of this cardiac conduction system stimulation pathway or pulse initiation point is the **sinoatrial (SA) node.** The SA node is called the **pacemaker** of the heart and it sets the pace or rate that the heart beats or pulses which is at the rate of about 70 to 80 beats per minute. This impulse is distributed to the right and left atrium as well as to the **atrioventricular (AV) node.** The AV node is also a pacemaker and it beats at a slower rate of 60 beats per minute. This AV node is a secondary pacemaker for the heart, a back-up for the SA node. The AV node conducts the impulse down amplifying the SA node nerve impulse. This conduction continues to the two large nerve bundles known as the **bundle of his or his bundle.** These two bundles are divided into the left and right **purkinje fibers** which are numerous branches spreading out and penetrating throughout all of the myocardium and all other regions of the heart providing a pulse for cardiac contraction. This stimulus contracts first on the right and left atriums then the right and left ventricles (Lub-dub) in this way it allows the blood to be pumped throughout the body. Now it is time to cover heart related problems.

Heart Disease and Failure (HDF)

Heart related medical diseases or failure do not just happen to the elderly individual but we do know that cardiac reserves decline as we become older. This decline can be due to age, infection or a disease process owing to the decrease in the immune systems. Although there may be other factors not related necessarily to age that are contributing causes to an assortment of cardiac and vascular conditions, such as, psychological and environmental stressors on the body which can impose physiological demands on the heart not only for the older generation but also for the younger generation. Dealing with the older adult, these demands can be more damaging triggering the heart to either increase in rate or slow the rate down or to cause an ineffective and irregular rate or rhythm. These stressors and risk factors can result in diminished function in activity of the heart causing circulatory volume flow changes, fatigue, shortness of breath, and changes in **tachycardia-rhythm.** Thickness in the walls of the vessels with aortic ventricle **stenosis** (narrowing) and valvular **sclerosis** (hardening) will cause systemic vascular resistance changes producing pressure against the walls of vessels to alter a person's blood pressure which can be part of the age dependent sequela. This age-related cardiovascular change will affect blood pressure with increase or decrease or even widening of the peripheral pulse rate. It can also have an effect on the quality; strengthening or diminishing feel of the outlying palpitation pressure, increasing the work load of the arteries, and the flow of blood to the right and left side of the heart. Much of this heart dyscrasia can be contributed to the loss of the peacemaker cell functions which can cause **arrhythmias** that can be noted on an electrocardiogram (EKG). **Baroreceptors** that regulate B/P which influence postural changes caused by hypotension (**orthostatic** movements), such as standing, sitting, bending, and movements of the head may cause dizziness and dizziness can lead to falls. The two most important arterial baroreceptors are located in the carotid sinus and the aortic arch.

When referring to heart disease one must not see the heart as the only fault in the system. It is everything we do and everything we eat and drink: it is how we live our lives; it is our activity or lack of. This sedentary way of life one lives is a prime offender or the demands of life that is wrought with unsolvable stressors that can riddle life's expectations and it is the environment we must endure which we may not be able to change which is a constant daily struggle in keeping life in some assembles of balance. Such is the lore of survival. So, you see, there are many factors involved with the maintenance of a strong heart, it is the constant upkeep of our health and that is a very tall order. The Center for Disease Control (CDC) and the United States Department of Health (USDH) understand this and are aware of these struggles. In August of 2015, the Center for Disease Control and Prevention updated their most common types of heart related diseases (https://ww.cdc.gov/heartdisease) and list 10 of the most common conditions. When reading this, one must keep in mind that the apoptosis or the normal aging and death of cells in the human body are going to happen. It is just the senescent or how these cells deteriorate or lose the power to grow that is important and how it relates to older adults. Are these conditions common-stances, that is, are they all age connected or not and can these changes be altered or slowed or better yet eliminated? These are the questions for another chapter. In the CDC update, there are 10 cardiovascular conditions named and this list will be used as a guide. Although, not all are specifically age related. I will go into them in a little more detail than the CDC:

Angina pectoris (AP) or ischemic chest pain can be a sign of coronary artery disease and is a discomfort of the chest that occurs in the area of the heart muscle when it does not receive enough oxygen-rich blood. Symptoms are pressure and a squeezing of the chest with associated radiating pain to the shoulders, arms, back, jaw, and neck. There are three forms of angina;

1. **Stable angina** which happens during above normal activities or during stressful, emotional, and mental demands.
2. **Unstable angina** that can occur at any time even at rest for no reason at all.
3. **Prinzmetal's angina** is a type of angina in which a coronary artery temporally narrows due to spasms. It usually happens when the person is at rest and it is often severe. It may be relieved by angina medication. Causes: stresses, smoking, and illegal drugs such as cocaine may trigger this event.

There are test that your doctor can use to determine if your heart is receiving adequate oxygen flow. Causes of AP, such as, this illustration is what an AP may look like.

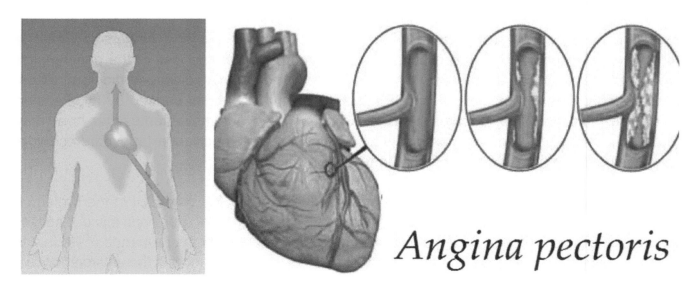

Angina pectoris

Aortic aneurysm and dissection are a ballooning/enlargement or weakening of the aorta. This ballooning or weakening of the aorta causes no systems until it ruptures. The cause can be related to high blood pressure, atherosclerosis, trauma, heredity, and other causes. Prevention is to decrease risk factors. **Aortic dissection** is a tearing and branching off of the inner layer of the aortic vessel (large blood vessel of the heart). Main cause of aortic dissection is high blood pressure. Other causes may be heredity, such as, **Marfan syndrome** (a genetic connective tissue disorder), trauma, smoking, cocaine, previous heart surgery, and others.

Arrhythmia is any abnormal changes in the sequence of electric impulse of the heart such as irregularity in rhythm or speed, be it fast or slow. In other words, your heart is just not beating normally. The more common abnormal arrhythmias can affect the atrial or ventricle chambers of the heart and can be life threatening. Some arrhythmias can be momentary as in the intake of foods, caffeine, over exercising, dehydration, and even minor stress can trigger this rhythm. Examples of some serious arrhythmias are atrial flutter, atrial fibrillations, and ventricular fibrillation. All arrhythmias should be noted and assessed by your physician.

Atherosclerosis and arteriosclerosis are basically two distinctly different concepts. Atherosclerosis is actually a form of arteriosclerosis and most people think that they are the same thing. Arteriosclerosis is a generalized term characterized by thickening and hardening of the walls of the arteries due to the accumulation of calcium and lipids, as well as, the loss of elasticity and narrowing of the artery limina. Atherosclerosis is more specifically a term for a disease in which the plaque builds up in the inner layer of the arteries and hardening of the arteries is/has taken place due to the same deposits as in the arteriosclerotic condition mentioned. Although the word is used the same, one means generalized condition and the other one is a disease process.

TERMS

- **Arteriosclerosis** is a general term describing any hardening (and loss of elasticity) of medium or large arteries
- **Arteriolosclerosis** is any hardening (and loss of elasticity) of arterioles (small arteries);
- **Atherosclerosis** is a hardening of an artery specifically due to an atheromatous plaque.
- **Atherogenic** is used for substances or processes that cause atherosclerosis.
- **Atherogenesis** is the developmental process of atheromatous plaques

From the American Heart Association. (Public domain)

Atrial fibrillation (AF) is an abnormal rapid irregular heart rhythm from the upper atria chambers. It may start off with palpitations, lead into light-headedness and progress to shortness of breath and chest-pain. Sometimes there are no symptoms at all and there are no real leads to follow up to this abnormal rhythm. Atrial fibrillation can lead to heart failure, kidney disease, dementia, and stroke. Some causes of AF are drinking too much, heavy caffeine use, exercising excessively, unlawful drugs, and inadequate sleep.

Cardiomyopathy is really a group of conditions that have an effect on the muscle of the heart enlarging it or causing it to become stiff. Many times, the underlying cause of cardiomyopathy remains a mystery but most cases can be discernible via a good medical history and laboratory test. Some causes are viral infections, uncontrolled hypertension, and a family history of the disease. Symptoms may be noted by shortness of breath, becoming easily fatigued, and swelling of the legs. This may progress to arrhythmia (irregular heart rhythm), dizziness, and fainting leading to an increase risk of cardiac death.

Congenital heart defects or (CHD) are the most common heart abnormalities that are present at birth. It has to do with the mal-formation of the heart and how blood flows through it and to the rest of the body. This mal-formation of the heart can involve the heart valves or holes in the walls of the heart's septum (wall that divides the left side of the heart from the right side). These defects can be minor to severe and the more severe ones are also called **critical congenital disease** and will need surgical intervention early in life. Many times this condition goes on noticed until the child participates in a sports activity.

Heart failure or (CHF) sometimes known as "congested heart failure" is the failure of the heart muscle to adequately pumping blood throughout the body and fluid starts to build up in the lungs, liver, and extremities. It is this failure of the heart muscle that occurs when the heart cannot pump sufficient blood to meet the needs of the body. The heart is just too weak to pump the blood throughout the entire body and retrieve it back to the heart. This is a chronic and long-term condition.

Peripheral artery disease (PAD) is an abnormal narrowing of the arteries that does not involve the heart or the brain. It is a common circulatory problem that usually affects the blood flow to the limbs. It is caused by atherosclerosis, the build-up of plaque within loom of the arteries narrowing the flow of blood to the limbs. This insufficient flow of blood to the limbs cause symptoms of leg pain or cramping when walking or exercising with systems stopping when one stops exercising or walking. At times it is accompanied by numbness and swelling to the affected limbs involved. This condition is called **claudication or intermittent claudication.** This condition is very serious and can lead to critical limb ischemia.

Rheumatic heart disease is a condition in which rheumatic fever due to bacterium streptococci pyogenes has permanently damaged the valves of the heart. It can be caused by strep throat or scarlet fever. There are two types of strep throats that are of major concern. The one that causes heart valve damaged is by an inflammatory infection of the A-Strep pyogenes that was poorly treated which then develops into rheumatic fever. This disease can affect any connective tissue not only the heart but also the joints, skin, and the brain. Rheumatic fever usually occurs in children around the age 5 to 15 but can occur at any age. Adults over 65 years old with health problems can be affected by the B-Strep pyogenes which can cause urinary tract infections, skin infections, blood infections, meningitis, and pneumonia. Both of these diseases are very rare in developed countries like the United States but do occur.

Other Health Related Changes in the Elder

Although this chapter is mainly on the cardiovascular system, it may be a good time to add these comments at this time. When one thinks about health it is about how one feels, looks, moves, thinks, visualizes life, and how one handles every day activities. This is correct but as we age there are changes in all of these important areas. The older one becomes a myriad of changes taking place internally as well as externally and these feelings, looks, thinking processes, how we move, our vision of life, the skin integrity, all our mental and physical youthful attributes and activities as well as all our internal organism become **different.** This goes for every system in the human body and although some of these systems have been discussed there are many that have not. There is a decline in our overall physiological reserve, our ability to continue to grow biological cells at the same rate as in our youth. This problem changes the way we use what is left and this poses a problem in trying to differentiate what is normal aging from the pathological aging processes, especially the one that impacts and interferes adversely with our ability to function properly our **ADL** (activities of daily living) and the one that affects our health.

Again, there are other organ systems that are declining and the rate of decline depends on the health and condition of the individual. For instance, the **pulmonary system** changes with age and this change is related to the respiratory system as it is involved with the heart. It has to do with the oxygenation and nutritional provision of the muscles that support the functions of respiration such as the intercostal muscles, the diaphragm muscles, and the many other muscles used for the purpose of increasing the diameter of the chest for the purpose of expanding the chest for air to enter the lungs to provide adequate breathing for our brain and cells; these breathing muscles begin to lose their elasticity, expandability, and strength. This causes the capacity and volume of air going into the lungs to be less than adequate with the inspired air to be reduced which is a decrease in ventilator volume. This is all related to the impaired chest muscles influencing the functional reserves of the respiratory system that affect the lungs inspiratory and expiratory breathing abilities causing endurance compromise and increasing one's respiratory breathing rate which can increase heart rate. You see how the human body is all connected and works as one complete structure.

Other human system's that normal aging affects is the **renal system,** the **urinary system,** and **reproductive system**. These last two systems are closely grouped together because they are anatomically in close proximity to each other and are referred to as the **genitourinary system.** The renal system refers to the kidney, the urinary tract, the ureters, the bladder, and the urethra. The reproductive systems for women affect the hormones and reproductive organs and for man it is the hormones and all this will also eventually become compromised by the aging process. Our **immune system** slows down and makes us more venerable to diseases. Seventy percent

(70%) of the human body's immune system lies within the **digestive system** this is why what you eat and drink makes such a great difference in your total health. The older we become the older all these systems become senescence affecting them all; the question is would this aging be within the normal aging of the human aging spectrum.

The most obvious and noticeable signs of the aging process and the one that people seem to care about the most is the winkles on their face, hands, and arms. This is the **integumentary system** or the skin tissue and is considered the first sign of aging. Some scientists think that the first real sign of aging is **alopecia** or balding but it is closely related to the changes that interfere with vision, balance or equilibrium. I think that wrinkles, alopecia, vision, and balance all start at the same time just that one may be more noticeable before the other. Looks and physical appearance become an issue and wrinkles on the face are the ones that truly bother us the most. As the body's external protector, the skin is the largest organ system of the body and it is exposed to the external environment on a 24-7-day period. It is an insulator and a shield against the outside atmospheric temperature, sunlight, harmful chemicals, a bacteria wall, as well as acting as a waterproof barrier. This amazing skin not only protects us from bacteria but protects us against infections and the skin makes vitamin D from the sun for our healthy bones. The skin has sensors which are nerve connections that allow the brain to be aware of what the skin touches and comes in contact with from the outside world and movement of the body is actually helped by this large organ system of skin sensors. There are seven layers of skin but what makes up the skin is collagen that provides firmness, elastin that provides elasticity and rebound, and **GAGs or glycosaminoglycan's** which helps in keeping the skin hydrated. The skin keeps the internal organs and muscles guarded and protected.

When it comes to natural aging, it takes place regardless of any outside environment and it usually starts at age 20 to 30. The normal cause is a reduced amount of collagen in our tissues so the skin becomes thinner and more easily damaged. There are fewer sweat glands and a reduction in oil glands secretion, elasticity slowly diminishes, and the GAG declines. Senescence or biological aging increases the cell death rate. This normal skin aging process is called the **intrinsic skin aging.** Added to the intrinsic aging is the **extrinsic skin aging** process and this is the result of the external environment aging or lifestyle aging. Ninety percent (90%) of this aging starts at the age of 30 and can be controlled and measured by the individual; smoking (tobacco or other), drinking (medication/drugs or alcohol), the sun (length of exposure time or high intensity exposure), stress (high stress situations), and air pollution. Many of these extrinsic processes can be balanced and controlled; added to this is good eating, Yoga, exercise, massages, and meditation which the Asians refer to as **Yin–Yang or universal balance.** This concept of Yin–Yang is that the amount of stress, movement activity, your job or any exertional effort, such as, exercise or just plain hard work should be balanced equally with the same amount of meditation, Yoga, or just plain relaxation with music, drawing or an activity that is soothing and relaxing to you: **'the balance of equal.'** Try it. This is why it is so important to maintaining one's physical, mental, emotional, social, and spiritual health.

Chapter 6

Dementia

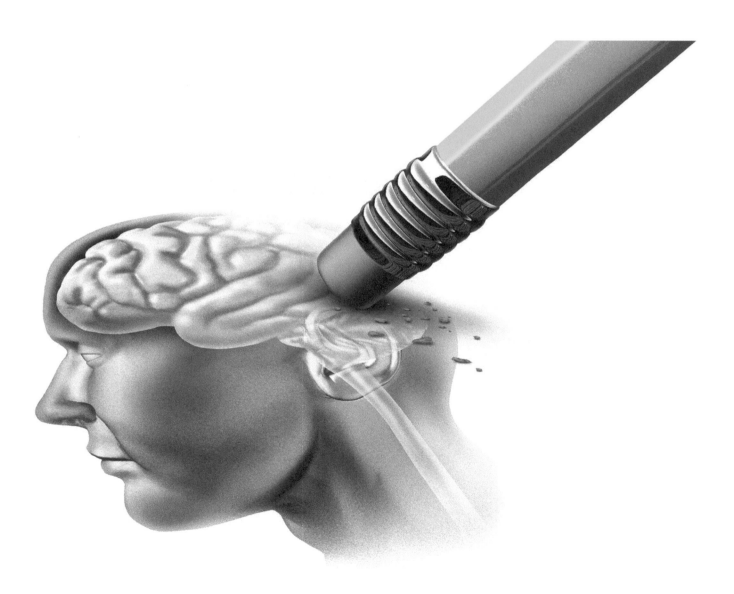

Contents in Chapter 6

Dementia

Maintaining one's health is 24-hour 7 day a week responsibility. It is not just eating well, making sure you are physically active, getting enough sleep, and avoiding as much stress as possible; it is a belief state of mind, knowing who you are, what you want, and having the drive to get there. It is a process of wanting to continually learn and educate oneself, finding good habits for a healthier lifestyle in the hope that they will guide you in the right direction and in maintaining the right attitude. This learning process refreshes the brain allowing oxygenated blood to flow unimpeded throughout the brain which allows the synapses to fire keeping the brain continuously engaged, active, and young. With this continuous motivation and effort, it gives one a reason to live and a will to stay healthy to reach and achieve the goals one wants to attain. When you add good breathing techniques, a reasonable amount of sleep time to this menu, life becomes much more tolerable in a more lifelong and therapeutic way. Why bring this up, because many of us choose the other paths, the path of less resistance, the one where drinking alcoholic beverages, smoking cigarettes, sleeping less, taking drugs not meant for healing or curing diseases or illnesses but to lose one's self in a fog of despair, wonder, and dissolution. This becomes a part of their life and controls their will; where a cigarette and/or alcohol becomes stronger than the will of the person smoking the cigarette or drinking the alcoholic beverage. This is O.K. if this is the road you choose or wish to travel and you select it with your mind and eyes wide open but where does this eventually lead you. What is not understood is that life does not owe you or any of us a damn thing, we owe life everything and when the brain gets these two ideological concepts off-stream, only chaos reigns. The body is the center or **the core;** it wants to survive and it will struggle to do so but with inadequate choices and self-protection are lowered and self-defensive mechanism becoming unreliable what is left is confusion to life's path which than becomes muddled and the body will not fully understand or succeed. The mind is a high-tech computer, whatever you put into it remains and the choices become scattered not only for the mind but for the body as well. This goes for all types of foods one eats, the quality of the oxygen taken in, the liquids we put into our body, medication/drugs we take, and any substances that can enter our internal environment. Yes, this also goes for desires, feelings, emotions, love, ideas, and hates. Does this have an effect on how the health of the brain works, how it sorts out important information and transmits the initiative to a response center and to our feelings; is it part of the inclusive health process of the body and mind link? This is all unknown to us at this time, that is, what really does drive the brain to work and tries to direct the body/mind/spirit on a specific path. There is an old saying "the heart beats in two ways in every person, one is with love and the other with hate; what you are can be summed up by the one that beats the most." You see, it all comes down to you. The body and mind are all one and the health of the mind is the same as the health of the body, the mental health follows the core and all conditions within its control.

What is Dementia?

Mental instability such as dementia is one of the human stigmata's that individuals may have to face when the body/mind don't coalesce. The fact is that we really do not know what the true root cause of dementia is, which by the way is also called **senility.** Dementia is a brain disorder associated with a disruption in communication that is connected with a group of symptoms such as those that affect memory loss, rational thinking, severe intelligence loss, and the inability to perform daily life activities. However, the loss of memory does not necessarily mean that you have dementia. As one becomes older, memory lapses or forgetful moments will happen. Age associated with memory lapses are considered to be a normal part of the aging process. This normal memory loss does not become worse over time but dementia memory loss **may** become worse over a few months. Alzheimer's disease (AD), a form of dementia are conditions in which one has trouble remembering things that affect their daily lives. That is when it becomes a watchful moment when he or she starts forgetting family member names, important events or conversations, forgetting words or important information, how to brush their teeth; this is when one needs to seek medical intervention. Hopefully one can catch these changes at its earliest stages. These memory losses are usually noticed by the spouse, friends, love-ones, and or close-net family members. Memory losses may be accompanied by changes in personality, such as, depression and anxiety, behavioral changes like agitation, hallucination, and paranoia.

Causes of Dementia

What is not always understood by many is that the health of the body **IS** the health of the brain and the health of the cardiovascular system is the health of the overall body. It's a circle that cannot be altered or broken. As stated, the body is a continuous circle of life and taking early preventive measures is very important to the overall health of the body. Is keeping a healthy mind and body going to help in reducing or preventing dementia? Well, scientists say yes but there is no positive conclusion to this question. It is within our scientific understanding that there are contributing risk factors that will enhance the causation of dementia. Researchers believe that there is a link between the risk factors and complications of the heart and the circulatory system that can lead to the progression of AD. Scientists at the U.S. National Institutes of Health have found that by reducing the systolic blood pressure to a range of 120 was affective in slowing down white matter lesions that have been linked to Alzheimer's disease. Many more of these risk factors have already been written such as the lack of exercise has been shown to increase the risk of dementia and people that eat unhealthy foods compared with those that eat a more **Mediterranean type diet** which are naturally grown foods, vegetables, and fruits. Using olive oil for salads and cooking, reducing the eating of red meats and substituting them for fish and white meat, wine is good in moderation (this I do not agree with because of the fermentation process and because the skin of the grape that has the resveratrol is thrown out), this has been shown to improve the health of the total body. As a meat lover, this would be a bit hard for me but it evidentially does work. What actually happens physiologically due to poor nutrition which may cause dementia is that the brain starts to lose nerve cells or neurons. The neurons are the brains sending and receiving centers that provide the pathways through which messages are transmitted. If the neurons in specific parts of the brain is damaged mainly around the part of the brain associated with memory and orientation due to poor nutrition; mainly the **hippocampus region,** Alzheimer's disease and dementia can develop. The hippocampus area is a storage area for memories and it seems to be a common area for AD and dementia to progress. There is no scientific, biological, or even a basic logical reason why this happens in this specific area and there is no known way at this time to reverse this process.

What we do know is that the brain of a healthy individual continues to grow neurons throughout their entire life and in a healthy brain this is a very delicate balance between the new growth of neurons and the dying neurons but for some reason new neurons just stops growing. This process is called **neurodegeneration.** Normally the protein waste or plaques that are produced around the brain break away and are eliminated but, in some cases, as in AD, the plaques build up in and between the neurons and the brain. This build-up structure around and within the affected neuron causes the neuron to lose its ability to function properly interfering with the synapse, that is, not allowing messages to pass between neurons in that particular area of the brain so that this segment begins to shrink leading to death of cells and weakening the function of the brain. This cell death is called **atrophy.** There are other reasons for dementia such as when blood vessels to the brain become damaged through a disease process or trauma. Hypertension can cause strokes and this can deprive the brain of oxygen which can damage and kill neurons at the site of the brain where the stroke developed due to lack of oxygen. Please be aware that not all strokes cause dementia; it depends on the area of the brain affected by the damage. This damaged site effects people in different ways with different symptoms. Having multiple strokes over time can be more concerning as this can result in what is called **Vascular Dementia.** There are other conditions that cause dementia like the **Lewy bodies** which is a plaque or protein found inside the neuron which affects the function of the neuron causing a Parkinsonian like syndrome and can also alter how dopamine receptors function and how it is produced and used in the body. This particular dementia is called **Lewy Body Dementia**. Be aware that some forms of dementia are reversible due to the fact that they are the side-effects or symptoms of other disease processes. Some forms of reversible dementia are:

> **Nutritional deficiencies such as vitamin B12**
> **Heavy metal poisoning**
> **The side effects of medication**
> **Thyroid gland that is underactive**
> **Some brain tumors depending on the location of the tumor**

Dementia Symptoms

Common signs of dementia have been stated but it is important to clarify the signs and symptoms in a more detailed and indistinct manner because these signs vary depending on the causes. The two most common signs are when cognitive abilities change and psychological changes take place which, as stated above, are memory areas and personality disorders. Dementia can also affect fine motor movements and coordination of these movements which can all be a part of the total interconnection of dementia syndrome. When one talks about signs of dementia, one must include the risk factors, such as, age that cannot be changed but there are many other risk factors that can be addressed. It is important, however, to know that dementia is **not** a normal progression of the aging process. There are cases that younger individuals in their forties and fifties and even younger as early as the 20's have developed dementia and even AD. One of these dementias that affect the very young is called Childhood AD or **Niemann-Pick Type C** which affects the cholesterol transport and fatty acids system in and around the cells. This leads to the build-up of fatty acid substances within the various tissues of the body including the brain leading to symptoms just like AD. It also shares symptoms with Parkinson's disease and Amyotrophic lateral sclerosis (ALS).

Complications of Dementia

Complications of dementia can radiate and affect the functions of many body systems. It can interfere with one's ability to perform every day daily hygiene activities, the ability to chew and swallow foods or water even saliva can cause lung aspiration and pneumonia, using the toilet becomes difficult and complicated due to memory lapse, and if left alone, dementia patients lose their ability to geo-synchronize and may wander away and get lost. In the late stages of dementia, the result of dementia can cause coma and even death. Most of these deaths are usually due to self-neglect and secondary condition such as poor nutrition, infections, and falls.

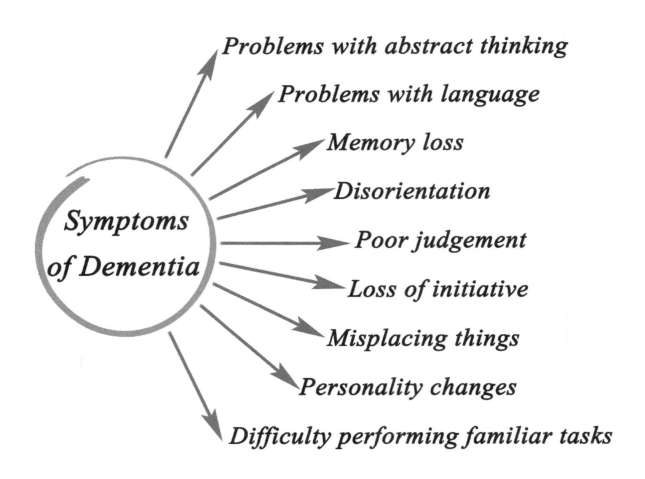

Problems with abstract thinking

Problems with language

Memory loss

Disorientation

Poor judgement

Loss of initiative

Misplacing things

Personality changes

Difficulty performing familiar tasks

Symptoms of Dementia

What is Alzheimer's Disease?

Alzheimer's disease (AD) **is a disease** and has been separated from the rest of the dementias because it is one of the most common irreversible brain disorders. For some reason AD seems to affect more females then males. There is on-going research as to why this disease targets women more than men and right now there is only a guesstimation. What we are aware of is scientists believe that this disease is a combination of genetics and a lifestyle that the individual is living. There is nothing one can do about one's genes but one can change how they live their life and this just may change the causes of this disease. The cause of Alzheimer's disease key word is that it is a **progressive** disorder due to the continuous wasting away of neuronal brain cells. This is a continuous decline and wasting away of neurons affecting the person's thinking, behavior, and social skills until all independent functions are disrupted. At this time around 5.7 million Americans have AD and this will climb to 14 million within the next 15 to 20 years. According to the **Mayo Clinic** a small percentage of Alzheimer's diseases are related to a mutation of three genes located in three different parts of the chromosome structure of the DNA which can be genetically passed down from one parent to the child and what is carried down has a high risk for the off-spring in developing AD. Please understand, just because you have one or more of these genes does not mean that you will develop AD. In fact, there are some with the gene that do not get AD and some without the gene do. One of these genes is called the **apolipoprotein E4 (apoE)** which are proteins that bind to lipids and form lipoproteins which is a particular type of lipids that is the major lipoprotein in the central nervous system and has been shown to be the major causation for dementia and Alzheimer's disease. There are a number of apolipoproteins; **apoA, apoC, and apoE** which have the same genomic structures and are members of the same multi-gene family that probably evolved from the same ancestry tree. Apolipoprotein is regulated in the intestines mainly by the fat content of the diet. Apolipoprotein is also controlled by the liver via hormones, alcohol, and various drugs. These apolipoproteins mentioned are not the only genes scientists have discovered that may play a part in AD. There are others. These other proteins that are produced in abundance in the neurons and the central nervous system that pathologies feel may have a link to the conditions related to dementia, such as, Parkinson's disease and Alzheimer's disease is **tau.** This protein called tau is said to help in the transportation network of nutrients to the neurons and the brain. In AD, this protein tau with the help of **amyloid-beta peptide** or protein begins to break down causing a twisted tangled blockage in the transport system and the **microtubules** or locomotive pathway of cells and specifically stopping nutrients and communication from reaching the cells of the brain. With this road block of nutrients the neurons die triggering a stoppage of messages to the brain and this cascading to other cells impacting the thinking processes and other mental and bodily functions. Scientists are still working to find out how tau and amyloid-beta peptides form these clusters and if it is these plaques that actually cause AD or is it a by-product of AD.

On-Going Research on Dementia and Alzheimer's Disease

Research into the origins, causes, and cures for dementia are being done by the **U.S. Department of Health and Human Service through the National Institute of Aging.** There is a private company called **"Tiaki Therapeutics"** in Cambridge, Massachusetts that has been theorizing and researching the causes of dementia and Alzheimer's disease. The company

Tiaki Therapeutics is supported by the **Dementia Discovery Fund (DDF)** which was set-up in October 2015 in London. Both organizations need funds and participants to continue their research. The **University of Texas, Southwestern Medical Center** is making great strides in the research on how to maintain healthy proteins before it becomes a toxic tau. This may help in the understanding and diagnosing of AD at an early stage and will be a great step forward in finding the many mysteries surrounding this disease. At **John Hopkins University,** research scientists have discovered ways to assess the biological and anatomical changes linked to Alzheimer's disease at least 10 years before symptoms actually appear and this research is continuing. In July 2019, in the Alzheimer's Association International Conference at the National Institute on Aging an announcement was made in a breakthrough in early detection of Alzheimer's disease via blood testing. Although not available to the public at this time due to privacy acts and worries which are a major concern at this time. Deciphering the causes of amyloid plaques and the tau tangles will give hope in the discovery and possible end to AD.

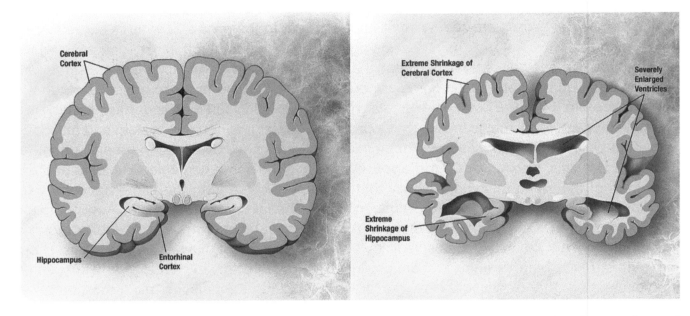

The National Institute of Aging – Dementia also called senility or senile dementia – Comparison of normal aged brain (left) and the brain of a person with Alzheimer's disease (right) with differential characteristics pointed out

New research is constantly going on, in fact, scientist is getting closer than ever to discovering what causes AD than ever before. It is thought that a bacterium called **Porphyromonas gingivitis** (P. gingivitis) may be one of the main culprits of AD but it may also be the cure. Research as shown that P. gingivitis which is a chronic gum disease may be the key to stopping and even reversing AD so says the World Health.Net, January 25, 2019 and Richard Hodes and Suzana Petanceska of the National Institute of Aging (NIA) in AARP March 2019 Vol.60-2 pf Pg.4 and this article continues to state that it has better tools to predicting new therapies that can help.

Unlike cancer, osteoporosis, and heart disease, it seems like there is not as much interest in this troubling condition. So far, dementia related illness continues to grow all over the world and will be a major concern as the older population also continues to increase. There is a greater need now for on-going research into the diagnosis, treatment, and the eventual cure of this wasting ailment.

Present Treatment for Alzheimer's Disease

It goes without thinking that if there is a reliable means to determine the probability of developing AD in a person, then it is without question finding a treatment, vaccine or medication modality too, at least, slow it down or to prevent it from becoming worse. Checking for genetic markers early in adult life may cause more questions, concerns, and confusion then needed. Scientists are aware that not all genes will actually cause this type of mutation. There are many different genes that have the potential to change a healthy cell to dementia or AD. Clinical test can help, such as, brain imaging may be useful in catching the disease at an early stage but it is important to understand that there is no single test that is going make a definitive diagnosis of dementia or AD. It is just a guide and it is up to you to find out how to use this information. Here are some diagnostic tools the physician will use to help in a prognosis:

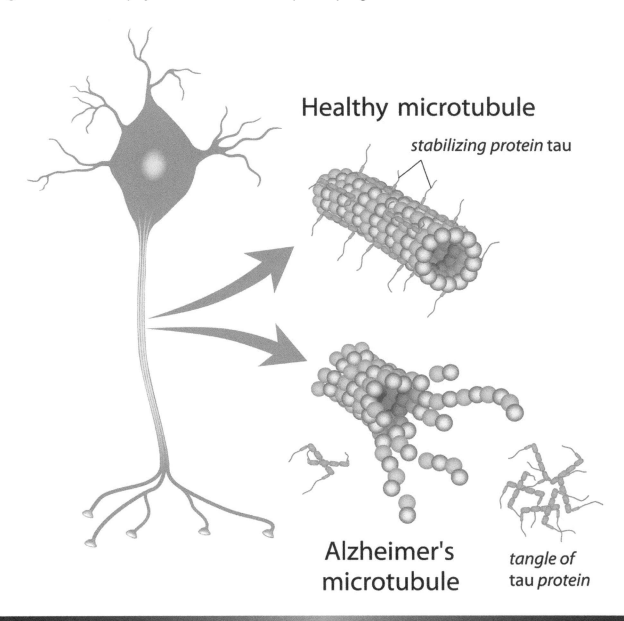

Healthy microtubule

stabilizing protein tau

Alzheimer's microtubule

tangle of tau *protein*

✓ **Medical history** especially the past family tree medical history which has significances and importance regarding current medical disorders or future medical possibilities or prognosis. It is a means of ruling out genetic indicators for other medical conditions, such as, cardiovascular problems, diabetes, H-B/P or hypertension, and many other markers of historical medical concern. This should include a history of past mental illness, neurological events, dementia or Alzheimer's diseases.

✓ **Physical examination** work-up will include checking the heart and lung sounds, blood pressure, blood and urine samples, and temperature and pulse check. The physician may find it necessary to perform other tests and make other assessments as per the gathering of all biological prognosis. The information gathered will also help diagnostication (diagnosis by conclusion) of issues related to dementia or AD.

✓ **Mental status assessment** may be done after the findings of all the assessments and this will evaluate neurocognitive and function abilities.

1) **MMSE or Mini Mental State Exam** is a questionnaire test to determine the individual's ability to follow simple commands, how oriented the person is to place, present time and date, his attention span and calculation skills, and his language and recall abilities. It is a 30-point test system that measures cognitive impairment that is used in medicine and other allied health services for dementia evaluation.

2) **Mini Cog** is a three-minute test that can increase detection of cognitive impairment in older adults. It requires the person to remember three names and remember them at a later time and to draw the face of a clock with all twelve numbers in the right place and a specific time on the clock.

✓ **Brain Imaging** is a way of determining if there is a structural deterioration that may be causing functional changes in the brain. There are a number of imaging technologies that can help map out the brain's biological parts by cross-section of the brain indifferent plains, sections, and depths of tissue loss. Some of these imaging technologies are:

1) **Computed tomography or CT** is an x-ray that combines a series of images from different angles around the body, in this case the brain, and it scans the brain creating cross-sectional images of the brain, that is, slices of the inside of the brain and soft tissues and processing the data producing an anatomic image in the slices of the brain.

2) **Magnetic Resonance Imaging or MRI** scan uses a strong magnetic field and radio waves to create detailed images of organs and tissues throughout the body; in this case the brain. It can diagnosis torn ligament to tumors and is very useful in the examination of the brain.

3) **Positron Emission Tomography or PET** is a nuclear medicine functional image device that is used to observe metabolic processes in the body, in this case the brain is used as

an aid in the diagnostication of any disease process. In the clinical diagnosis of the brain, it can be of help in determining the disease factor or the causes of various dementias.

There are many other tests that can be used in determining memory decline but these are just a few. These tests cannot give a conclusive diagnosis of dementia or AD, it may help in showing the why in memory loss and other potential memory problems. It may also show stages of progression of the memory loss.

Alzheimer's: Drugs Helpful in Managing Symptoms

There is no medication that will stop Alzheimer's disease but there are medications that will manage the symptoms in the hope of prolonging independence. Alzheimer's drugs cannot slow down the progress of the disease and they do not work for all who take them. By the time dementia or AD symptoms start to appear, much of the neuronal damage to the regions of the brain affected has happened and the loss of memory due to this damage has already taken place. Early detection is really the key strategy to research scientists in the hope of stopping this disease. According to the Mayo Clinic, there are two drugs that have been approved by the **Food and Drug Administration** for specific stages of Alzheimer's mild, moderate, and severe and they are based on stages of memory loss.

Cholinesterase inhibitors boost the amount of acetylcholine, a neurotransmitter that is responsible for alertness, memory, thought, and judgment to the nerve cells preventing the breakdown of acetylcholine in the brain. These medications eventually will lose their ability as the disease progresses. There are three types of cholinesterase inhibitors approved:

- **Donepezil (Aricept)** – approved to treat all stages and taken as a pill.

- **Galantamine (Razadyne)** – approved to treat mild to moderate stages and taken as a pill.

- **Rivastigmine (Exelon)** – approved to treat mild to moderate stages of Alzheimer's disease and can be taken as a pill or skin patch.

- **Memantine** – is approved to treat mild to severe Alzheimer's disease and works to regulate the activity of glutamate which is a chemical used in sending and receiving messages from one cell to the other in the brain. It can be taken as a pill or syrup.

Research on Alzheimer's Disease

In a Harvard Health Publication dated April 2011, researchers have been studying the idea of combining the use of two strategic medications aimed at different targeted areas in the hope of slowing the progress of memory loss in regard to the causes of dementia and AD. These targeting medication ideas are specifically geared towards the tau tangles and the amyloid-beta peptides. Memantine with another cholinesterase inhibitors for example may be more effective in slowing down cognitive decline than those patients taking just the one cholinesterase. This mixed medication cocktail is still being studied to determine the effectiveness of this type of treatment. There are more than 80 medications currently under investigation in the treatment of Alzheimer's disease at this time. There is hope that a medication or a combination of medications can be found to slow down the progress of cognitive loss and/or halt this disease's destructive course that kills brain cells. At the **University of Central Florida Neuroscience Division, Professor Kiminobu Sugaya** is researching the stem cell concept for the re-vitalization of brain cell neurons and/or replacement of those cells that have degenerated due to the damaged brain cells as in Alzheimer's disease, Parkinson's disease, and ALS (Amyotrophic lateral sclerosis). Other research facilities and universities are also looking into stem cell technology for therapy in the hope of finding ways to stop this debilitating disease. Great strides are being made in this particular field and should be watched closely in the future.

I must inject this word of concern at this time and that is that we should not overlook the known risk factors, such as, maintaining a healthy lifestyle by exercising or increasing your level of activities as importance for all healthy endeavors especially for those with dementia or AD. This increase in activities can be as simple as a walk around the block, tai chi, some aerobic exertion, doing things in pottery class or in the garden, and taking up Yoga class as long as these activities are above your normal daily routine. A healthy and planned diet which means reducing red meat and eating more fish and chicken, vegetables, nuts, whole grains, beans, and fruits are good and are all your friends, avocados are great and the use of olive oil may be a life saver for you. This is all part of the Mediterranean diet or a part of any healthy diet. Less meat and more fruit and vegetables would work just as well. There is so much more that is recommended by the Mayo Clinic and their recommendations should be looked up.

Chapter 7

Nutrition and Longevity

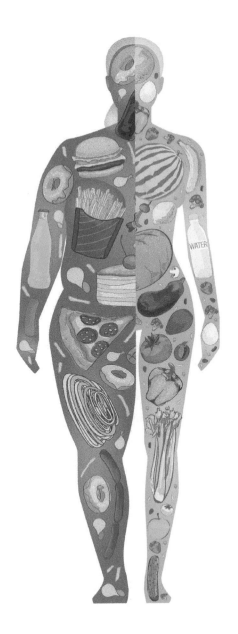

Contents in Chapter 7

Nutrition and Longevity

Nutrition is the number one topic throughout the world and it is the one thing that is essential for the continuation of life. It is concerned with the foods that we find to eat and the way these food substances are used to nourish our body. This nourishment of the body has a great physiological impact on the way that it affects the responses in side our body's and how it breaks it down. These chemicals that are in this food substances we have eaten are for the purpose of cell physiology, bio-cellular growth, tissue repair processes, metabolism, and energy production within our cells to ensure life's continuation. There are a number of definitions of nutrition but as is stated above and broken down here into simpler words: nutrition is concerned with how the foods we eat are broken down and used in the body. The nutritional need starts at the beginning of conception and continue throughout old age until death. Health is dependent on meeting the basic biological human needs of the body and when health is maintained so is life's expectancy maintained and extended.

Regaining Control of Our Health

There is no secret in staying healthy or maintaining one's health, it is just that it takes too much of an effort to go through the process. Everyone knows what to do, what's good and what's not-so-good, it's just that we don't want to make and/or take the time and energy to concern ourselves with it. I went through that stage; the idea is in the brain but the will to actually do it is absent; I get it. The will and the tenacity have not been nurtured or brought to importance yet. Finding the path is hard and when you read about it in books and magazines they really are all saying the same things but have new names for what is basically the same view, for instance, Holistic Health, Wellness, Being Whole, Total Wellbeing, Holistic Practice, and a myriad of other concepts and words but if you look and read these powerful words and ideas it all comes down to the same few elements;

1. **Have a well-balanced diet,**
2. **Increasing your daily level of activities,**
3. **Reducing your stress as much as possible,**
4. **Try to get an adequate amount of sleep.**

The reality is that people live in a dynamic world and in different socioeconomic statuses that are culturally diverse in their ideas and with their own ethnicity, milieus, beliefs, and needs. Maybe religion or a spiritual belief plays a role and we all know that the will of the individual plays a major rule as to maintaining one's health. It is really nice to see these beautiful people in magazines exercising, doing Yoga or meditating and one can only wish to be like them but when you finish reading the magazine and it is put down the dream is over you come back to reality, you're still you. It is no mystery that having a strong belief in an idea or one's self can trigger a willingness that can activate a hidden strength that will attract you to want to do or be something special. That is the beauty of living. That special something could be that faith that inspirers the will to perform better, develop skills faster or just a lifelong activity of maintaining a good sound healthy program of habits. Being healthy entails every aspect of every cell in the body not just a state of health in mind and body but also the fact that you have made every effort to do what you can to stay and/or maintain your overall health and fitness goals. It is that word **effort** that is missing from these magazines and healthcare periodicals that should be highlighted and should form the foundation of health goals first and foremost importance and the key in the word **"mind and body." Wellness means all the EFFORTS made in maintaining a healthy and physically fit state-of- mind and body.**

Health and Good Nutrition

The best way, and many think the only way, to be healthy and to maintain one's health is through a healthy diet. It is hard to say no to this because it is in a large way partly the truth. A healthy diet controls the physical and mental needs necessary for life. Albeit, for every country and every culture they have their own differences when it comes to foods and boundless drinks and then you add the spices and herbs that are used it becomes a guesstimation as to what is a healthy food or drink to put into the body. Other countries and cultures have healthy children and adults just like all more modern societies and cultures. What foods really constitutes or is classified as a healthy food?

Nutrition or the foods we eat, I think, have to have a number of qualities; they have to be readily available, be masticatable, go through the process of ingestion, then digestion, followed by absorption of the digested substance. Next, the food must be able to go through the human metabolism of the digestion which is absorption of the substance, through assimilation, and then finally elimination of the non-usable waste products from the body. That's pretty straight forward. According to the 'Merriam Webster Dictionary' **nutrition** means "the process of eating the right foods so you can grow properly and be healthy." Again, the foods that all cultures and all nations are eating must be sufficient to sustain the growth of the human species cells and to be able to maintain the human existence for health and life. This means that these foods contain the basic nutritional elements necessary for growth and life regardless of what the food is that are being eaten. If that's the case, the food must have the basic nourishments required or substances necessary in its complex form to promote human development regardless of what social culture one lives, such as, **macronutrients and micronutrients.**

Macronutrients

When talking about the foods we eat it comes down to the quality of nutrients we're putting in our body. This means the worth of the substances that the body needs for nourishment of which are essential for the growth, development, and maintenance of life. The basic nutrients necessary for which the body needs in large amounts are **carbohydrates or sugars, lipids or fats, proteins or amino acids, and water.** These four nutrients are needed in quantities sufficiently enough for the physiological and biochemical demands and functions of the body and are referred to as macronutrients. You might say that macronutrients are the fundamental life's intrinsic and indispensable essence of all living things on this beautiful planet we call earth. What we hopefully derived from these macronutrients is the necessary seeds of life itself.

Carbohydrates or starches – These nutrients provide the energy or fuel for the body as does lipids or fats. Proteins can also function to provide energy or fuel for the body but it is not its primary function.

Proteins or amino acids – These nutrients promote growth and development of muscles, tissues, organs, and for continuous growth and repair of tissues as required.

Lipids or fats – These nutrients are a storage form of concentrated energy or fuel for the human body and are the backups for the carbohydrates as an available energy source.

Water – This is truly the **food of life** and is a substance that is transparent, tasteless, odorless, and an almost colorless chemical that is within all living organisms. It is the main ingredient in every living thing and in human it is the primary catalysis for metabolism, absorption, and transportation of nutrients to all the cells in the body. Water is a universal solvent and most revered food substance on the planet. There is no life without water.

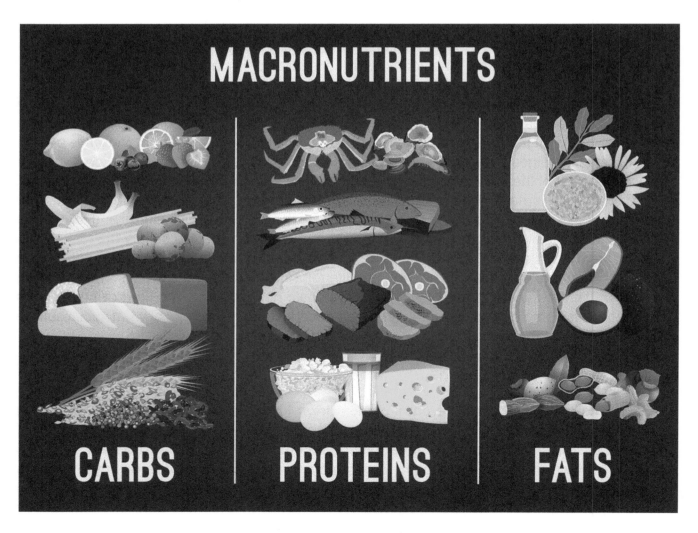

Micronutrients

Micronutrients are the roots of the seeds of life and is what comes from the macronutrients. These roots or nutrients are **vitamins, minerals, and trace elements** needed in small amounts but basic necessities for the health of the body. These micronutrients are not used as fuel, they are used as a nonprotein compound that is necessary for the function of an enzyme and are essential for the binding properties to proteins so that a biochemical reaction can work and when put together with a protein are called co-enzymes. Most co-enzymes are vitamins such as Vitamin B-2, B3, and C needed in small or trace amounts for normal metabolic enzyme function. **Enzymes** are mostly proteins and a few are catalytic RNA molecules called ribozymes. An enzyme is a substance produced by the living organism that acts like a catalyst to bring about a specific biochemical reaction. **Catalysis** is a process that speeds up a chemical reaction without being consumed or altered in the process and is of immense importance to the body. Enzymes such as amylase, pepsin, DNA polymerase are considered the catalyst of the body and vitamins play a key role in its function. Vitamins are necessary for enzymes to function and help it to complete their activities. Vitamins are non-protein organic molecules that facilitates the catabolic action of its attached enzyme. **Adenosine triphosphate or ATP** is a co-enzyme that provides energy to the muscles of the body to perform work.

Minerals are elements that cannot be synthesized in the human body. They come mainly from the foods we eat plants, animals, and from the water we drink and the air we breathe. There are 21 essential minerals or elements: 7 major minerals that play a role in electrolytes and 18 trace minerals. There are also 13 essential minerals 5 non-essential minerals and all of these minerals the human body needs to stay healthy.

Minerals and trace elements are necessary for the growth of the human body and needed to preserve the integrity of the body. They have to be taken in to the body through one's diet and are part of the matrix and the structure of the body. These 21 minerals and some trace minerals are required to support the human biochemical processes within our body and serve for structural, functional, and electrolytes stability for the maintenance of life. As with the vitamins, some minerals such as calcium, potassium and magnesium are needed in larger amounts than other minerals.

MAJOR MINERALS
Calcium (Ca)
Phosphorus (P)
Sodium (Na)
Potassium (K)
Magnesium (Mg)
Chloride (Cl)
Sulfur (S)

TRACE MINERALS

Essential	**Unclear**
Iron (Fe)	Silicon (Si)
Iodine (I)	Tin (Sn)
Zinc (Zn)	Cadmium (Cd)
Selenium (Se)	Arsenic (As)
Fluoride (Fl)	Aluminum (Al)
Copper (Cu)	
Manganese (Mn)	
Chromium (Cr)	
Molybdenum (Mo)	
Cobalt (Co)	
Boron (B)	
Vanadium (V)	
Nickel (NI)	

Vitamins are an essential organic molecule that is needed by the human body in small amounts for metabolism function and most be obtained through the diet. There are 14 known vitamins: four are fat-soluble and 10 are water soluble vitamins. Some vitamins are needed in larger amounts then other vitamins because of the health needs of the body.

Fat soluble vitamins

A – Retinol

D – Cholecalciferol (not a true vitamin it's a hormone)

E – Tocopherol

K – Koagulations vitamin

Water soluble vitamins

B_1 – Thiamin

B_2 – Riboflavin

B_3 – Niacin

B_5 – Pantothenic Acid

B_6 – Pyridoxine

B_7 – Biotin

B_9 – Folate

B_{12} – Cobalamin

C – Ascorbic acid

Choline (considered a B vitamin)

Carbohydrates in a Nutshell

Carbohydrates are the fuel for the cells of the body and this food or nutrient comes in many forms but they all must fulfill one basic need in order for it to be of service to human biological life needs. It must be broken down into a fuel form and source or glucose that will provide energy, structure, function, and the biochemistry necessary for the human body. Carbohydrates are the primary fuel source for this necessary energy and power that all organisms need to sustain life and promote the health needs to do their work. A plant, through the energy of the sun's solar rays enables them to manufacture carbohydrates within their own cell walls through a system called **photosynthesis.** The soil provides the minerals the plants need to maintain plant development. Plants store these carbohydrates and minerals that humans need within their plant cells and as we eat these plants and through digestion, absorption, and metabolic function, we are able to use this by breaking down the plant's nutrients, into the necessary starches and minerals needed for energy and growth. Plants are the major food source of caloric energy in the form of carbohydrates, vitamins, minerals, and fiber for humans.

Energy Production System

There are three factors in providing basic fuel to the body:

1. 1. Change the basic fuel to refined fuel designed for human needs.
2. 2. Carry this refined fuel to places that need this fuel or energy.
3. 3. Burning this refined fuel in areas designed to use it.
4. 4. Elimination of the unused substance and byproduct of digestion.

In America, more than half the total calories are in the form of plant carbohydrates and they are relatively low in cost, easily obtainable, and are easily stored.

Vitamins at a Glance

Vitamin	Function	Sources and Stability	Dietary Reference Intake	Disorders Related to Deficiency	Disorders Related to Toxicity
Retinol and (vitamin A and Provitamin A)	Protects vision pigment; promotes resistance to infections and growth of healthy epithelial cells.	Fish, liver, dark oranges, yellow and red fruit and vegetables. Heat stable. Destroyed by exposure to light.	Men: 900 mcg Women: 700 mcg Upper adult limit: 2000 mcg	Alcoholism (by precipitating zinc deficiency), celiac disease, fat malabsorption, and respiratory disease.	Cheilitis (dry lips), nasal, eyes, and skin mucosa, hair loss, nail fragility, bone pain, gingivitis, hepatomegaly, and ascites
Cholecalciferol (vitamin D3) Ergocalciferol (vitamin D2)	Facilitates calcium absorption from the intestine and maintenance of phosphorus levels in blood. As antioxidants, prevent oxidation of unsaturated fatty acids and maintains the integrity of cell membranes.	Fatty fish, eggs, liver, and fish liver oils. Available mostly in artificially fortified products, such as, milk, yogurt, breakfast cereals, and bread. Very stable, but pure cholecalciferol is destroyed by high temperatures and humidity. Most stable form is obtained by encapsulating vitamin D3 within a protective matrix.	Adults: 51-70 yr. 10 mcg (400 IU) Adults >70 yr. 15 mcg (600 IU) Upper adult limit: 2,000 IU	Rickets, depression, abnormal functioning, and premature aging	Excess or deficiency can cause abnormal functioning and premature aging.
Tocopherol (vitamin E alpha, vitamin E beta, and vitamin E gamma)	Maintains the integrity of the cell membrane.	Vegetable oils, leafy green vegetables, and whole grains (wheat germ). Destroyed by heat, light and oxygen.	Adults: 15 mg Upper adult limit 1,000 mg	Sterility, cystic fibrosis.	No known toxicity.

Vitamin	Function	Sources and Stability	Dietary Reference Intake	Disorders Related to Deficiency	Disorders Related to Toxicity
Quinones (vitamin K1 and vitamin K2)	Formation of several blood clotting factors in the liver. Synthesized by bacteria in the large intestines.	Green leafy vegetables and some fruit, dairy products, meat, and eggs. Moderately stable to heat and reducing agents. Destroyed by acids, alkali, light, And oxidative agents. Best derived from food sources only.	Men: 120 mcg Women: 90 mcg Upper adult limit: N/A	Women: 90 mcg Upper adult limit: N/A	Thrombogenesis, hemolysis, and increase risk of jaundice (rare).
Thiamin (B1)	Breaks down carbohydrates	Fortified cereals, pork, and navy beans. Destroyed by heat and baking soda.	Male: 19-70 yr. 1.2 mg Female: 19-70 yr. 1.1 mg	Beriberi, "pins and needles" sensation.	No known toxicity.
Riboflavin (B2)	Supports energy metabolism.	Meats, poultry, nuts, peanuts, cereal.	Male: 19-70 yr. 1.3 mg Female: 19-70 yr. 1.1 mg	Mouth sores and inflammation.	No known toxicity.
Niacin (B3) Niacinamide	Supports energy metabolism.	Meats, poultry, nuts, peanuts and cereal.	Male: 19-70 yr. 16 mg Women: 19-70 yr. 14 mg Upper adult limit: 35 mg	Pellagra	Flushing and redness.
Pantothenic acid (B5)	Synthesizes coenzymes important for fatty acid, and energy metabolism.	Beef, poultry, potatoes, and vegetables.	Adults: 5 mg	Rare	No known toxicity.
Pyridoxine (B6)	Amino acid metabolism.	Liver, fish, poultry, fruits, and whole grains.	Adult: 19-50 yr. 1.3 mg Male: 50-70 yr. 1.7 mg Female: 50-70 yr. 1.5 mg Upper adult limit: 100 mg`	Microcytic hypochromic anemia	Weakness, numbness

Vitamin	Function	Sources and Stability	Dietary Reference Intake	Disorders Related to Deficiency	Disorders Related to Toxicity
Biotin (B7)	Fatty acid synthesis and metabolism, gluconeogenesis, and amino acid metabolism.	Liver, nuts, and eggs.	Adult: 19-50 30 mg	Rare	No known toxicity.
Folate (B9)	Metabolism of amino acids and synthesis of DNA; cell division and development t of neural tubes in fetuses.	Fortified cereals, spinach, broccoli, black and pinto beans, orange juice, and potatoes. Extremely vulnerable to heat.	Adult: 400 mcg Upper adult limit: 1,000 mcg	Neural tube defects in fetuses; macrocytic anemia.	No known toxicity but can mask a B12 deficiency.
Cyanocobalamin (B12)	Folate absorption, synthesis of myelin.	Liver, meat, eggs, and milk.	Adult: 2.4 mcg	Pernicious and macrocytic anemia.	No known toxicity.
Ascorbic acid L-Ascorbic acid vitamin C)	Maintains iron and makes it available to the hemoglobin, and the metabolism of certain amino acids.	Fruits and vegetables, especially oranges, grapefruits, Papaya and strawberries. Destroyed by light, heat air, iron and copper.	Men: 90 mg Women: 75 mg Upper adult limits: 2,000 mcg (77,000 IU)	Scurvy (weakened connective tissue, lesions, impaired wound healing, and poorly formed collagen).	Nausea and diarrhea (rare).
Choline	Maintain the structure of and integrity of cell membrane, synthesis of acetylcholine, and neurotransmitters.	Milk eggs, liver, and peanuts.	Adult: 700 -1,000 mg	Liver damage.	Low blood pressure, fishy body odor, sweating, excessive salivation, and reduced growth rate.

Minerals at a Glance

Mineral	Function	Source	Dietary Reference	Disorders Related to Deficiency	Disorders Related to Toxicity
Calcium (Ca)	Bone and tooth formation, blood clotting, muscle and nerve action, and metabolic reaction.	Milk and milk products, yogurts, cheese, and ice cream, bok choy, collards, broccoli, kale, and turnip greens	Adult: 19-70 yr. 2,000 to 2,500 mg	Tetany, various bone deformities, and increase bone fragility.	Increase kidney stones, interference with absorption of iron, zinc, phosphorus, and magnesium.
Phosphorus (P)	Bone formation, energy metabolism, and acid base balance. Serves as a partner to calcium.	Milk and milk products, meat, fish, and eggs. It's found in all animals and plant cells	Adult: 700 mg	Rare	No known toxicity.
Sodium (Na)	Body water balance, acid base balance, muscle action, nutrient absorption.	Animal products, such as, milk, meat, and eggs. Vegetable products, such as, carrots, beets, leafy greens, and celery.	Adult: 19-50 yr. 1.5 g Adult: 50-70 yr. 1.3 g Adult: over 71 yr. 1.2g	Acid-base balance disorder and cramping.	Hypertension and water build up in the tissues.
Potassium (K)	Works with sodium in water balance and many other metabolic functions, muscle action, insulin release, and blood pressure.	Unprocessed foods: oranges, bananas, broccoli, leafy greens vegetables, meats, whole grains, and milk products.	Adult: 4.7 g	Can occur through prolonged vomiting and diarrhea. The use of diuretic drugs, severe malnutrition, and surgery.	Weakened and/or stoppage of the heart. Poor muscle tone, and breathing difficulty,
Magnesium (Mg)	Widespread metabolic functions and is found in all body cells. Muscle action, basal metabolic rate, and protein synthesis.	Nuts, soybeans, cocoa, sea foods, whole grains, dried beans and peas, leafy green vegetables.	Men: 19-30 yr. 400 mg Women: 19-30 yr. 350 mg Men: 31> yr. 420 mg Women: 31> yr. 320 mg	Rare	No known toxicity.

Mineral	Function	Source	Dietary Reference	Disorders Related to Deficiency	Disorders Related to Toxicity
Chloride (Cl)	Helps control water and acid bases balance in digestion. Assist red blood cells during respiration.	Sodium chloride (table salt)	Adult: 2.3 g	Rare	Only known cause is dehydration.
Sulfur (S)	The structure of hair skin and nails, metabolic function, vitamin and collagen structure.	Meats, eggs, milk, legumes, cheese, and nuts.	Not stated.	Rare	No known toxicity.

What are Carbohydrates?

There are numerous types of nutrients and all are organic compounds found in living things. All organic compounds contain carbon which is the most abundant element in humans. Other frequently found elements in humans are hydrogen and oxygen. Carbohydrates are composed of these elements **Carbon (C), Hydrogen (H), and Oxygen (O),** and is abbreviated **CHO.** Carbohydrates are also known as starches, saccharide or sugars. Deoxyribose is a sugar that functions as a building block for DNA. **Saccharine** is a single unit sugar and saccharides are called a **monosaccharide.** Carbohydrates are classified according to their number of single sugar units. **Monosaccharide and disaccharides** are called **simple carbohydrates** such as raw sugar, brown sugar, corn syrup, fructose and high fructose syrups, glucose, and sucrose. Even fruit juice concentrate is considered a simple carbohydrate. Complex compounds of saccharide units in long chains are called **complex carbohydrates.** The complex carbohydrates have more nutrients and more fiber which help it digest slower and facilitates better weight management control. It is better tolerated for diabetics and will help manage their sugar spikes after a meal. These complex carbohydrates are called **polysaccharides or starches and dietary fiber.**

Monosaccharides

Glucose is a form of sugar that is circulated in the blood and is the primary fuel for the cells. It is not found in the diet as such, except in corn syrup and processed food.

Fructose is found mainly in fruits or honey and it depends on the degree of ripeness as to the amount of fructose.

Galactose is usually found in the diet but comes mainly from digestive milk sugar or lactose.

Disaccharides

This carbohydrate is composed of two sugar units linked together. The three most basic disaccharides are:

Sucrose = Glucose + Fructose – This is common table sugar and is made from cane or sugar beets.

Lactose = Glucose + Galactose – This is sugar in milk, found in mammary glands as lactose and not found in plants.

Maltose = Glucose + Glucose – Not found as such in the diet. It is derived from the digestive breakdown of starches.

Polysaccharides

This carbohydrate is a complex chain of many single sugar units. This nutrient includes starch, glycogen, and dietary fibers.

1. **Starches** are the most important and significant polysaccharide carbohydrates in the world and the most important source of carbohydrates for energy in the body. Starch has a more complex structure then simple carbohydrate sugars. They are found in grains, fruits, legumes, dairy products, vegetables, nuts, and seeds.

2. **Glycogen** is found in animal muscle tissues; this is called animal starch. Once digested by humans, the animal starch is fermented in the body and is crucial to the body's metabolism and energy balance. It is stored in the liver and muscles and is constantly being recycled and broken down into glucose for energy as needed.

3. **Cellulose or dietary fiber** has no energy value but is very important in the diet. Dietary fibers are composed of glucose units but cannot be broken down by the human digestive system. Dietary fiber does add bulk to foods and helps move foods along the digestive track through a movement called **peristalsis** and at the end forms feces for elimination. Some forms of dietary fiber absorb water and thus slows the movement and emptying of waste products down providing fermentation material and also work in the colon so that the good bacteria can do their work. There are three major types of this dietary fiber **cellulose, non-cellulose polysaccharides, and lignin.**

The Functions of Carbohydrates

As stated, carbohydrates are the basic fuel supply for the body. Its primary goal is to meet the energy fuel needs of the body at a rate of 4kcal/g. This means 4 kilocalories per gram or 4,000 calories per gram of body weight. Fat is also a fuel but the body only needs a small amount of dietary fat. Glycogen is a polysaccharide of glucose and is a storage form of this energy reserves for the body. It is primarily made and stored in the cells of the liver and the skeletal muscles and just like triglycerides and adipose tissue they all supply the vital backup fuel for the body's needs. The total amount of carbohydrates stored in the body, including blood sugar and glycogen is relatively small and has to be replenished constantly. This requires the liver to continuously make and supply glucose to the working muscle especially those of an athlete and physically active individuals.

Dietary Reference Intake for Carbohydrates, Sugar, and Fiber

Calculating your DRI calories and grams of carbohydrates are recommended.

1. Keep track of everything you eat for one day. Using a Food Composition Table Chart, calculate your daily food intake. This is your total energy intake.
2. Total energy intake = __ K-calories.
3. Multiply your total energy intake by .45 and .65 to get the number of calories (Kcal) from carbohydrates (CHO).

   __ Total kcal X 0.45 = __ kcal
   __ Total kcal X 0.65 = __ kcal

Example: 3000 total kcal X 0.45 = 1,350 kcal
          3000 total kcal X 0.65 = 1,950 kcal

Your carbohydrate kcal range that you have taken are between 1,350 and 1,950 kcal/day.

Anatomy of Lipids or Fats and Their Function

If one sees a fat cell under a microscope one would see a bulbous egg-shaped sphere that has a cell membrane. In this spherical membrane there is a nucleus, mitochondria's, droplets of stored ATP with at least 3 fatty acid molecules depending on the type of cell (more on this later). The functions of lipids are the basic storage of potential energy for the body. It is also the structural component of the cell walls. Fats or lipids are the second group of organic compounds that are essential to the human organism. Lipids composition is the same as the elements that carbohydrates are made of; carbon, hydrogen, and oxygen but the ration of oxygen and hydrogen is not the same. Not all lipids are easily soluble in water but are soluble in alcohol, chloroform, and ether. There are many forms of lipids some are in solid form and some in liquid form and can be as; phospholipids, carotene, vitamin E, vitamin K, vitamin D, and prostaglandins.

Classification of Fats

1. **Lipids** – are the overall name for the chemical group of fats.

2. **Triglycerides** – are esters of glycerol and three fatty acids that are made up of the same chemicals as carbohydrates; carbon, hydrogen, and oxygen. As a group, these fats are called glycerides because glycerol is attached to the fatty acids' molecule. Most natural fats, either animals or plants, have one glycerol molecule and three fatty acid attachments and so it is given the name triglycerides or neutral fats. Triglycerides are the most common fat in the body. Calories that are not used or needed in the body are converted to triglycerides and stored in the fat cells. When energy is needed it is released from the fat cells by the body's hormones. Triglycerides are under your skin and around your organs and act as insulation for the body. Triglycerides are also in your muscles, liver, and are used as backup fuel for the body.

3. **Fatty Acids** – is the main building block of fats and are classified by the chain length, short, medium or large. This depends on the number of carbons attached to it. There are two characteristics of fatty acids which relates to its single bonds of carbon chains. <u>**Saturation fatty acid chain**</u> contains all its single hydrogen bonds of carbon and <u>**unsaturation fatty acids**</u> do not. There are specific bodily needs for fats that are necessary for life; essential or nonessential fatty acids needed for use in the body.

   ➤ **Saturated fatty acids** are those fatty acids that contain all the material that is needed and is capable of holding. Saturated fatty acids have the full complement of hydrogen bonds it can hold which makes it heavier, denser, and more solid, whereas;

   ➤ **Unsaturated fatty acids** do not have this full complement of hydrogen bonds. This means that it is less heavy, dense, and solid.

      A. **Monounsaturated fatty acids** are missing one hydrogen spot or bond. Example: olives and olive oil, peanuts and peanut oil, avocados, canola oil, almonds, pecans, coconut oil, palm oil.

      B. **Polyunsaturated fatty acids** are missing two or more unfilled hydrogen spots or bonds, vegetable oil, safflower, corn, cottonseed, and soybean.

   ➤ **Essential or Nonessential Fatty Acids**

      A. **Essential fatty acids** are needed in the body and without them create specific deficiency diseases. The body cannot manufacture these essential fatty acids so they must be obtained from the diet. The only known essential polyunsaturated fatty acids needed by the body that must come from foods we eat are **linoleic and linolenic fatty acids.**

B. **Nonessential fatty acids** are fatty acids that the body is capable of producing in the body, such as, saturated fatty acids, monounsaturated fatty acids, and cholesterol; therefore, these fatty acids are not needed by oral intake so there is no set intake requirement for these fatty acids.

4. **Lipoproteins** – a combination of fats (lipids) and proteins which is the major vehicle of transportation in the blood. It is carried in the blood for needed nutrition. Lipoproteins contain triglycerides, cholesterol, and other material, such as, fat soluble vitamins. A lipoprotein's relative load of fats and proteins are determine by its density.

> **Low density lipoprotein (LDL)** has a higher fat load which carries fat and cholesterol to the cells.
> **High density lipoproteins (HDL)** have a higher protein load and carries free cholesterol from the tissues to the liver for breakdown and excretion.

Cholesterol

Cholesterol is not really fat. It actually is related to a group of chemical substances called sterols or modified steroid and is a vital substance in human metabolism that occurs naturally in all animals and plant tissues. Since the body manufactures cholesterol, there is no biological dietary need for the intake of cholesterol consumption.

A Little More on Cholesterol

Cholesterol is an organic molecule. It is a type of lipid that is an essential part of the constituency in the total biochemistry of the body that is required for all plants and animals. Cholesterol is chole=**(bile),** stereos=**(solid),** ol=**(alcohol)** and is a sterol or modified steroids necessary for the proper membrane permeability and fluidity of all cells. It is a form of lipid that is needed within the cells, outside of the cells, and is required for steroidal function that is also needed by the body to make hormones. It is essential in the conversion of bile acid in the gall-bladder and for the stabilization of fat-soluble vitamin, carotene, D, E, A, and K. This element is very important and necessary for intracellular transport, cell signaling, and nerve conduction within the human body. Cholesterol is made by the cells but the greatest amount is made in the liver and it makes all the cholesterol it needs for the physiology function of the human body.

Not only do animals make cholesterol but plants also make cholesterol called **phytosterols.** Knowing that cholesterol is made from animals and plants, the question is; how much cholesterol does the body need? Well, cholesterol is calculated by the weight of the individual. If you weigh 150 lbs., the typical total body cholesterol synthesis is 1g or 1000mg per day for a total body content of 35g primarily located in the cells of the body. This means your body does not need to ingest any extra cholesterol but typically, the daily diet intake of additional cholesterol, in United States, is 200-300mg. Although high cholesterol levels are a great risk factor for heart related ailments, the intake of dietary cholesterol has little to no effect on the levels of cholesterol or on your risk of heart disease. High cholesterol is usually caused by life style factors, diet, and the genes as well as medical conditions or by some medicines. Please keep in mind that the ingested cholesterol is poorly digested and absorbed and the body compensates for any increase in cholesterol absorbed by reducing cholesterol synthesis in the liver so high diet intake of cholesterol above the body's need and production of cholesterol will accumulated and be stored in the body's tissues. Higher amount of cholesterol may be produced by the body and this can greatly contribute to elevated cholesterol levels but this is not the norm. Low density lipoproteins (LDL) molecules are the major carriers of cholesterol in the blood and each molecule contains 1,500 molecules of the cholesterol ester. High density lipoproteins particles are thought to be the transport of cholesterol back to the liver for excretion or to other tissues that use cholesterol to synthesis hormones in a process known as **reverse cholesterol transport (RCT).** That is why it is better to have HDL because it actual helps to break down LDL.

Treatment Options for High Levels of Low-Density Lipoproteins

There are a number of medications called **statins** also known as **HMG-CoA reductase inhibitors** that are said can reduce or lower cholesterol in the body. Statins are a class of medications that act to lower or reduce the levels of fats including cholesterol and triglycerides in the human body by **inhibiting the enzyme** called **HMG-CoA reductase,** which plays a role in the production of cholesterol in the liver. So far, there are at least 7 different statins on the market today that are classified as a statin medication but there are several combination preparations of statins and other agents also available. Your physician will determine if you are a candidate for one of these statin treatment modalities. This will be determined by your family history and your medical history. Please keep in mind that a good diet regiment, exercise, especially aerobic can be of great help in lowering cholesterol in the body.

The Function of Fats as Energy and Essential Nutrients

Fats serve as a fuel for the body just as carbohydrates do, but fats also are an important form of insulation for the body and a storage form of fuel because excess carbohydrates are converted to stored fats. As stated above, fats also carry triglycerides for added energy and fat-soluble vitamins which aids in absorption in the body.

Body Fats

Adipose tissue are fats that is stored in various tissues of the body. It acts as padding and cushion support for vital organs, generates energy when needed, and regulates the body temperature. Women have more adipose tissue cells than men. There are two basic types of fatty tissues; brown fatty tissue (BAT) and white fatty tissue (WAT). BAT contain smaller lipid droplets and numerous mitochondria's that give it its brown appearance. BAT generates heat better than the WAT. This heat generation is called **thermoregulation** and it is the primary function of BAT. WAT main function is the energy storage for the body.

Animal Verses Plant Fats

Saturated fatty acids predominantly come from animal sources whereas plant fatty acid foods are mostly monounsaturated and polyunsaturated fatty acids.

Visible and Invisible Fats

Obvious fats are plain to see, such as, butter, margarine, separated cream, salad oils and dressings, lard, and visible fat on meats. It is easy to control the visible fats in your diet. Fats that are less visible and hard to control in the diet are cheeses, cream in homogenized milk, egg yolk, nuts, seeds, olive oil, avocados, and lean meats. The dietary requirements for fats should not exceed 20% to 35% with 10% provided from saturated fats and 300 mg/day from dietary cholesterol. If your goal is to lose weight, it is a good idea to record your intake of nutrients taken on a one-day period of time times three days. Divide this by three so in this way you can visually see what you are actually putting into your body. Using a nutritional chart, you can calculate your calories, amount of proteins, and fats consumed. Based on this information, you can determine a course of action you may need to take.

Prostaglandins (PG)

Prostaglandins or PG are a large group of membranes that are associated with lipid compounds and may have diverse hormone effects. They are in almost every tissue in the human body. They contain 20-carbon atoms, 5-cardon rings, and may have different purposes even different effects as well as reverse activities on different body tissues. PG is produced in all nucleated cells in the body. Their purpose is to modulate and help hormones response when it comes to menstruation, secondary abortion, and are involved in inflammatory response, platelet aggregation, and regulating the temperature in the body.

Proteins

Proteins are a much more complex structure then carbohydrates or lipids. This third group is immense in both structure and complexity and are composed in units called amino acids. Amino acids are composed of carbon, hydrogen, oxygen, and nitrogen atoms with sulfur and phosphorus sometimes present. Protein is responsible for most of the structure of the body cells and is important for the biochemistry and function for all the enzymes and muscle contractions.

What is the Function of Proteins?

These amino acids are joined together in unique chain sequences to form specific proteins types. A peptide bond joins amino acids together to form two or more amino acids or chains. Amino acids can form together in two's or in hundreds. Hundreds of amino acids are linked together to form a specific protein. Large complex protein molecules can be subject to mutation or malformation which can lead to protein building mistakes such as **Alzheimer's disease** in older adults or **PKU (phenylketonuria)** which is associated with neurological deficits in infancy).

As stated, protein compound is made up of carbon, hydrogen, and oxygen that make up carbohydrates and fats, but protein also has 16% nitrogen which is not in the other two. A protein or amino acids are reassembled after digestion in a specific order to form a variety of tissues e.g., collagen in connective tissue, myosin in muscles, hemoglobin in red blood cells, and digestive enzymes or hormones. The average size adult contains between 10kg to 12kg of protein with the largest quantity located in the skeletal muscles. Protein content remains remarkably stable in the human body and there are very little to no reserves of protein stored in the body.

Classification of Amino Acids

There are 20 common amino acids that are necessary to human life and health. These amino acids have three classifications; **indispensable (essential), dispensable (nonessential), and conditionally indispensable (conditionally essential).**

Indispensable Amino Acids

These nine amino acids cannot be left out of the diet because the body cannot manufacture them in sufficient quantities. The remaining 11 amino acids, under normal circumstances, can be synthesized by the body as long as the nine indispensable amino acids are present.

Dispensable Amino Acids

Under normal circumstances, these five dispensable amino acids can be synthesized by the body via the other indispensable amino acids provided that the necessary amino acids and enzymes are present.

Conditionally Indispensable Amino Acids

The remaining six amino acids, under normal physiological conditions, can be synthesized by the body but if the metabolic demands are not available, these amino acids must be consumed in the diet. Example: the body can make cysteine as long as methionine is available. If methionine is not available then cysteine must be consumed. Stress, illness, and genetic disorder can render amino acids conditionally indispensable.

Protein Balance

Body proteins are continuously breaking down into amino acids with a release of energy and a by-product of nitrogen. This process is called **catabolism.** Rebuilding (re-synthesizing) into tissue proteins is called **anabolism.** Nitrogen is the by-product in the amino acids chain. It is removed and converted into **ammonia (NH_3)** and excreted as urea in the urine.

Nitrogen Balance

Nitrogen balance depends on how tissue protein is being maintained in the human body. The dietary intake of proteins in foods is measured by the amount of nitrogen that is excreted in the urine. If the protein balance taking in equals the nitrogen excreted in the urine (6.25g of protein equals 1g of urinary nitrogen) the body is said to be in nitrogen balance.

Positive Nitrogen Balance

If the body takes in more nitrogen (protein intake) than it excretes in the urine, this is called positive nitrogen balance. This storage of nitrogen is because the body is building more tissue than it is breaking down. This occurs during infancy and childhood growth, pregnancy and lactation, and illness and malnutrition when the body is being built back up. This also can be seen during the course of body building and other strenuous exercises.

Negative Nitrogen Balance

This means that the intake of nitrogen (protein) into the body is less than it excretes and is a negative nitrogen balance. It is due to an inadequate amount of protein intake and is breaking down more tissue then it is building up. This is seen in **kwashiorkor, hyperthyroidism,** fevers, burns, protein deficiency, and other wasting diseases. This causes the loss of muscle tissues, impairment of body organs, and susceptibility to infection. This can also be seen in the aging population and can be due to dementia and AD (malnutrition in the elderly).

The Purpose of Proteins

The fundamental structure of every cell in the body is protein. Lean muscle mass accounts for about three-fourths of the protein in all the dry matter in most of the body tissues, excluding bone and adipose fat. The primary purpose of proteins is to repair the wasted or damaged tissues and the building up of new tissues and is central to the biochemical machinery that makes cells work. This process slows down as we age.

Amino Acids and Health

There are 20 common amino acids that are necessary to human life, as stated, the health of the body and they have basically three different classifications, to repeat, these proteins or amino acids classifications; **indispensable (essential), dispensable (nonessential), and conditionally indispensable (conditionally essential).**

Indispensable, Dispensable, and Conditionally indispensable Amino Acids		
Indispensable	**Dispensable**	**Conditionally Indispensable**
Histidine	Alanine	Arginine
Isoleucine	Aspartic Acid	Cysteine
Leucine	Asparagine	Glutamine
Lysine	Glutamic Acid	Glycine
Methionine	Serine	Proline
Phenylalanine		Tyrosine
Threonine		
Tryptophan		
Valine		

DRI and the Recommended Dietary Allowance (RDA)

Carbohydrates is the primary fuel source for the body's energy Kilocalories (4 Kcal) and is assisted by fat (9 Kcal) as stored fuel. In time of need protein may furnish additional fuel as a back-up source. The available fuel factor of protein is 4 Kcal/g. The Dietary Reference Index or DRI has set the recommendations for proteins as a percentage of total Kilocalories (Kcal) for consumption for children and adults at 10% to 35% of their total dietary intake from proteins. The RDA has set for men and women at 0.8g of high-quality protein per kg of desirable body weight per day (0.8 kcal/kg body weight per day) and for heavy training 1.2 to 1.8g/kg per body weight. The use as an energy source of protein is dangerous and destructive to the organs and cells of the body. From the recommendation of the DRI (10% to 35%) and the standards of the RDA for both men and women (0.8g per kg) let's calculate the protein needs:

If you calculated that you consumed 2200 calories (Kcal). Use a "Food Log" form to calculate your daily intake. One day per page.

    2200kcal X 0.10 = 220 kcal per day from proteins
    2200kcal X 0.35 = 770 kcal per day from proteins

    220 kcal ÷ 4 kcal/g = 55 g of protein per day.
    770 kcal ÷ 4 kcal/g = 192.5 g of proteins per day

The protein needs of a female 5'6" and weighs 270 lbs.

    Convert pounds into kg.
    (2.2 lb. = 1 kg)
    270 lb. ÷ 2.2lb/kg = 122.72 kg
    122.72 kg X 0.8 g/kg = 98.18 g of protein per day

Manufacturers' Claims for Amino Acids	
Amino Acids	**Claims**
Arginine	Improves immune function, increases tissue creatine levels, increases release of insulin and growth hormone, leads to fewer gastrointestinal problems, and improves performance.
Aspartate	Improves energy metabolism in muscles, reduces amount of fatigue causing metabolites, and improves endurance performance.
Glutamine	Improves immune function (fewer colds), hastens recover exercise, improves performance, and leads to fewer gastrointestinal problems.
Ornithine	Increases growth hormones and insulin release, stimulates protein synthesis and reduces protein breakdown, improves performance.
BCAA	Provides fuel for working muscles, reduces fatigue, improves endurance, reduces muscle protein breakdown.
Tyrosine	Increases blood concentrations of catecholamine's (epinephrine & norepinephrine), improves fuel mobilization and metabolism during exercise.
Tryptophan	Increases the release of growth hormones, improves sleep, decreases sensation of pain, and improves performance.
Taurine	Delays fatigue, improves performance, facilities faster recovery, leads to less muscle damage and pain, leads to fewer gastrointestinal problems, scavenges free radicals.
Glycine	Increases phosphocreatine synthesis, increases sprint performance, and improves strength.

Please be careful of the many claims made regarding the use and benefits of different proteins. These are just some claims that the makers of the protein products are claiming the amino acids can do for the body. Research from an independent authority is still out and until proven, be aware.

A Little On BCAA

Branch-Chain Amino Acids (BCAA) which is **leucine, isoleucine,** and **valine** is the most abundant amino acids in the human body and accounts for 35% of all the amino acids in the human muscular system. Your body does not make these amino acids so they must be in the foods you eat and are called "essential" amino acids. Milk has 8g of protein in the form of casein and whey and so one drink of an 8oz glass of milk you can receive all the amino acids required for an active sports person as well as all the BCAAs and all the essential proteins needed. The reason why I am bringing this up is because BCAA is the most popular nutritional supplement sold today but this can be satisfied by one 8oz glass of milk. There is no evidence to prove that in higher quantities of BCAA that it can reduce net protein breakdown, reduce fatigue, and enhance performance via the central nervous system mechanism. Until this is proven through scientific research stay with the proven 8oz glass milk before and after an exercise and save your money.

On nutrition needs, the recommended ratio of nutrients to support a physically active person can be summed-up as following:

Carbohydrates 45%-65% of total kcal
Fats 25%-30% of total kcal
Protein 10%-35% of total kcal

In discussing macronutrients and micronutrients there is an understanding that we are presenting the most basic knowledge for better awareness of the facts regarding carbohydrates, lipids, proteins, vitamins, and minerals. There is so much more that is not presented, for instance, where does one draw the line between how much carbs, protein or fats one should take for the different degrees of physicality or activity one does. Is it better to exceed the recommended calories or vitamins for a very active individual in hope that they may be needed and the body can eliminate the unused nutrients? When it comes to minerals there are 94 naturally occurring minerals or elements on the Periodic Table and our body needs just a small portion of these natural elements. Are there other elements that our cells need but are not showing up in microbiology research or are we still on this learning curve and just do not understand all that we need too at this time regarding the biological elements in life?

According to the NIH National Institute on Aging all nutrients are important for all ages but the key vitamins and minerals needed for people over the age of 51-70 are **vitamin D** at least 15mcg (600IU) each day but not more than 100mcg (4,000IU). Over 70 years 20mcg (800IU) but not more than 100mcg (4,000IU) and the best source is fish, fish liver oils, fortified milk and milk products, and fortified cereals. **Vitamin B$_{12}$** at least 2.4mcg every day from meat, fish, poultry, milk, and fortified cereals. Some over 50 may need supplements and fortified foods. For **calcium** 51-70 years of age, 1,000mg to 1,200mg a day as you get older for men and for women 1,200ng a day. For both men and women do not exceed 2,000mg each day. When it comes to **magnesium** women need 320mg a day and men need 420mg each day. Dietary fiber as green leafy vegetables, legumes, nuts and seeds, and grains contain this mineral. Water also has these minerals as does fortified foods and cereals. To get an adequate amount of **potassium** for a person 51 years of age and older you need at least 4,700mg every day. Milk, potatoes, coconuts, dried apricots, lentils, is rich in potassium. For more information on Vitamins and Minerals contact the Office of Dietary Supplements National Institute of Health ods@nih.gov or www.ods.od.nih.gov. I am sure that there are many more mysteries still to be discovered when it comes to nutritional needs of the human body and for the healthiest nutritional benefits for our aging population. After all of this, I can only wonder why adding a little more protein to the diet is not a good thing to do for the aged population. Senior citizens may want to take a tip from body builder's and make whey protein shakes a regular part of their diet. According to researchers at McMaster University, drinking a whey-based shake boosted the physical strength in a group of men at the age of 70. A drink of Ensure, Boost, Nutriment, or even an extra 8oz glass of milk should be a good practice for good health. Milk, by the way, contains 8g of protein with all the essential amino acids, fats, and carbohydrates the body needs in just an 8oz glass. No other food contains all three basic food groups and with added Vitamin A and Vitamin D it becomes the food of the Gods. I like it with chocolate and sometimes strawberry syrup.

Nucleic Acid

The nucleic acids are a compound in the nuclei cells. These are large organic molecules composed of building blocks just like proteins that are made up of carbon, hydrogen, oxygen, nitrogen, and phosphorus of which there are two principle kinds; **deoxyribonucleic acid (DNA) and ribonucleic acid (RNA).** As we have stated, they are the basic units of protein which are amino acids but the basic unit for nucleic acids is the nucleotides. **Nucleotides** are organic molecules that serve as the units for forming nucleic acid polymers (units bonded together) as DNA and RNA. Nucleotides are the building blocks of nucleic acid. They are composed of 3 sub-units of molecules: nitrogenous base or nitrobase, 5 carbon sugars (ribose or deoxyribose), and at least one phosphate group. Each molecule of DNA or RNA is composed of repeated units of these nucleotides which consist of these three basic parts;

1) **Nitrogenous bases** that are found in DNA's - adenine (A), thymine (T), cytosine (C), and guanine (G). Adenine and guanine are double-ringed structures (helix) collectively called purines and thymine, cytosine and uracil (U) are smaller single ringed structures called pyrimidines. They are united as base-pairing to form the helix structure. RNA uses uracil rather than thymine and RNA are single-helix structures,

2) **Pentose sugars** or five-sugars of ribose or deoxyribose and,

3) **Phosphate groups** are a chemical compound made up of a phosphate and four oxygen atoms when connected to a molecule. Phosphate groups are the sugar-ring that connects the nucleotides of the nucleic acid to the backbone of the phosphate band end-to-end into a long chain creating a single double helix.

The chemical components of the DNA were known since 1900 but the organization of its actual structure was not known until 1953. This structure or model was proposed by biochemists James Dewey Watson and Francis Harry Compton Crick after exhaustive investigations. This structure consisted of two long chains of nucleotides with the complementary based pairs that twist to form a double helix that look like a spiral staircase and the connection is held together by weak hydrogen bonds. The hydrogen bonds hold the complementary base pairs together such thymine and adenine which form the genetic coding. All life is based on this genetic coding and its arrangement and connection of these essential bondings.

Adenosine Triphosphate (ATP)

Adenosine triphosphate is a molecule and is a part of the **phosphate** group that provides immediate energy source for every cell in the human body. The body stores this energy for various cellular activities. As stated, this ATP molecular structures consistency is a three-phosphate group (PO_4^{3-}) and an adenosine unit composed of adenine and the five-carbon sugar ribose. Because of its total amount of usable energy when it is broken down by hydrolysis (water molecule) it is considered a high-energy molecule. Once ATP is broken down by hydrolysis, it liberates a large amount of energy which is utilized by the cell for cellular functions. This cellular function or activity removes a phosphate group leaving a molecule called **adenosine diphosphate (ADP).** This breakdown of ATP to ADP is called a **catabolism** (breakdown of a cell and the release of energy). ADP can be converted back to ATP by replenishing the phosphate group. This is done by the decomposition reaction in the cell, in particularly with the glucose. Glucose is completely broken down or metabolized in the cell's activity and leaves carbon dioxide and water and the energy released in this process is used to reattach a phosphate group to the ADP which resynthesizes ADP to ATP. In this way,

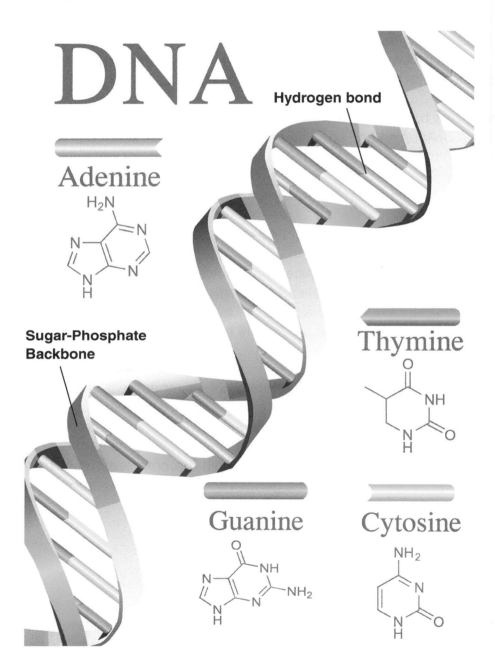

ATP is constantly being manufactured for cell use. When ADP remanufactures and replenishes the phosphate group and resynthesizes the ATP, it is called **anabolism** (the building-up in the body of complex chemical compound from smaller simpler compounds).

Cells and Cell Physiology in Aging

In order to introduce cell physiology as it relates to aging in its direct terminology, I have added it to this chapter. The human body as in all living things are composed of cells. Aging is the progressive failure of these cells' homeostatic adaptive response. Cells contain the DNA and the RNA for growth and health and repair of the human body. It also contains the power house or mitochondrion that fuels these cells keeping them active. When the cells organelles begin to age, they start to become dysfunctional, diminish in quantity, and/or fail. In some way it changes the structure, function, and purpose that make the cells on a whole work. This makes it more vulnerable to diseases that is brought about by the internal and external environment and by stressors.

As mentioned, the characteristics of aging like graying of hair, loss of teeth, loss of hair, unsteady gait, vision changes, decrease in muscle mass, and an increase in weight are all signs of this slow deterioration brought about from various functions and activities of daily living, vis-a-vis with this total environment. This gradual deterioration affects the kidneys, hormonal balance, and the ability to adjust to temperature changes, dieting adjustment, oxygen use, and the internal body metabolic function. Causes are due to an overall decrease in the number of properly functioning working cells in the body especially cells in the brain. Aging tissues cells also change the collagen fibers that give strength to the muscle tendons that start to decrease in collagen quality and number. This is called intrinsic skin aging. This, likewise, happens in the arterial walls which are responsible for the deposits of the fatty material that starts to adhere to the interior aspects of the arterial walls causing **arteriosclerosis**. Decreased collagen in aging also affects the elasticity of the blood vessels itself making it thicker and less elastic with a greater ability for the absorption of calcium within the vessel walls hardening the walls itself and this condition is called **atherosclerosis.** Atherosclerosis and arteriosclerosis many times are used interchangeably but they mean different conditions. Yes, arteriosclerosis can mean any general term or condition involving the vessels and it is more than likely you have atherosclerosis but until you are actually diagnosed and told what you have by your doctor you should wait until you receive the doctor's results. Arteriosclerosis is more of a general term used for many vessel dyscrasia of the vascular system where as atherosclerosis is a specific disease process of the vessel. As you can see apoptosis affects all cells and different body parts at various times and degrees. Cells will continue to grow a number of times but once they reach their limit as to the number of times they have reproduced; senescence will be inevitable. This number depends on the individual's health and age, the environment, and many intertwining genetically programed events.

How To Eat Healthy Chart

Stress Management
Activities

Stress will cause you to eat more food than needed. Lower your stress by exercising at least 30 minutes a day.

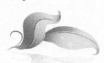

Quantity
Calories

Track the amount of calories you eat. An average meal should be between 400-600 calories. This includes 3 meals a day and 2 100 calories snacks.

Water
Sugarless Hydration

Drink water with every meal. Water keeps your body systems working normally. Avoid soda and other chemically made drinks.

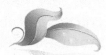

Meals
5 Meals a Day

Eat 3 meals and 2 snacks per day. Eating 5 times a day will keep you from feeling tired. Plan your meals to avoid impulsively eating

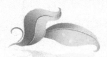

Breakfast
Don't Skip Breakfast

Eat a healthy breakfast every morning. Breakfast provides the energy you will need to start your day.

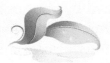

Saturated Fat / Trans Fat
Read Labels

Read the labels on the foods you eat. Eat foods with less than 3 grams of saturated fat per serving. Protein, saturated fats and trans fats are the most available type of nutrition in the average city.

Fiber
Stay Full

Eat foods high in fiber like whole wheat, oatmeal, vegetables, nuts and fruits. High fiber foods keep you feeling full longer.

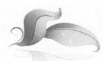

Salt
Read Labels

Read the labels on the foods you eat. Remove salt from your table. Use spices to enhance the flavor of your foods. Also use fresh onions and garlic.

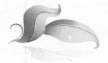

Chapter 8

Foods and Nutritional Supplements
for the Elderly

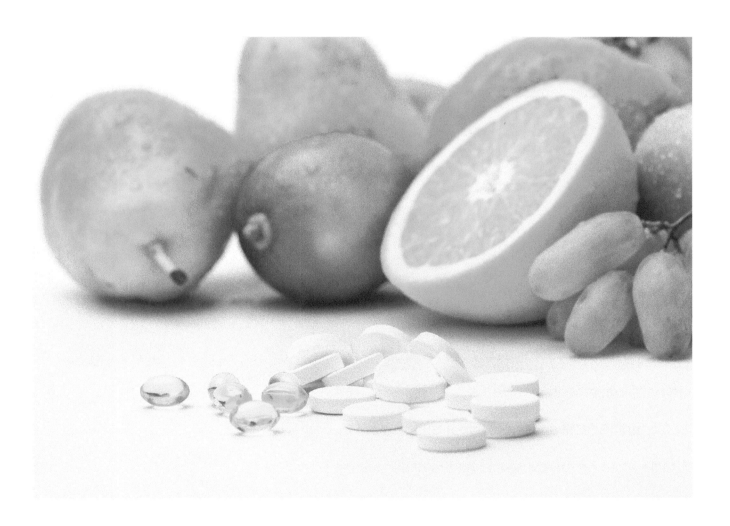

Contents in Chapter 8

Foods and Nutritional Supplements for the Elder Adult

Although we have covered some aspects of nutritional supplements, such as vitamins, minerals, proteins, and fats it is important to understand why certain nutrients play a more valuable role for the older population. As time takes its toll and the aging process in humans' marches on so does the different needs of the body. Your daily meals and the one-a-day vitamin may not be enough to maintain the body's needs in accommodating its nutritional requirements. There are extreme pros and cons regarding the need for any nutritional supplemental needs but this is assuming that all older adults are eating a well-balanced diet or understand what a well-balance diet even looks like or supposed to be. In this, I can honestly say that most "ABSOLUTELY DO NOT." We all understand the importance of eating well and having a balanced diet in maintaining and staying healthy as one ages but the fact is, it just does not happen anywhere in this beautiful world and the sooner we face this the better. We must pay attention to the facts and fit the pieces into these needs in a real-life event. Before talking about nutritional supplements, let's talk about how we can improve our love one's and our own nutritional and social needs. Most of these were already covered and worth repeating:

- **Encourage healthier food choices.**
- **Have foods used for snacking chosen from a healthier variety.**
- **Good tasting healthy foods will go over much better.**
- **Encourage exercise, even a simple jogging in place at home or a walk around the block is great.**
- **Have planned social activities.**

Consider eating various types of protein choices and include these foods in your choices like lean meat, fish, beans, peas, and add whole grain cereals, breads, crackers, rice or even pastas which are all good choices and include a dairy product such as milk, yogurt or cheese, especially those fortified with Vitamin D. When talking about healthy snack choices, it can be as simple as apple slices, grapes, bananas, yogurt, berries or peach slices, almonds or walnuts, orange slices, cottage cheese, and I am sure you can think of other food items. Bananas for instance, are a great snack and can help older adults maintain a healthy weight balance, in fact, it may help them loss a few pounds due to the fiber content. Ten percent of the banana is fiber and if you combine a light to moderate amount of exercise or physical activity with this it will enhance the senior's health diet. It is important to stay hydrated with beverages that are healthy. Much of the body's hydrational needs will come from the foods that are eaten. More on hydration later. There is a food chart outline that is very good and I hope it will help one to understand the nutritional value of certain food sources. This **Therapeutic Food Chart for Health** can be shared with others.

Missing Nutrients in Older Adults Diet

It is important to know that as we age so does the number of needed calories as well as the body's ability in absorbing key nutrients. Our ability to taste and to smell foods also

Therapeutic Food Chart for Health at a Glance

Apples	Protects the heart	Prevents constipation	Blocks diarrhea	Improves lung capacity	Cushions joints
Apricots	Combats cancer	Controls blood pressure	Saves the eye sight	Shields against Alzheimer's	Slows the aging process
Artichokes	Aids digestion	Lowers cholesterol	Protects the heart	Stabilizes blood sugar	Guards against liver disease
Avocado	Battles diabetes	Lowers cholesterol	Helps to stop stroke	Controls blood pressure	Smooth's the skin
Bananas	Protects the heart	Quiets a cough	Strengthens bones	Controls blood pressure	Blocks diarrhea
Beans	Prevents constipation	Helps hemorrhoids	Lowers cholesterol	Combats cancer	Stabilizes blood sugar
Beets	Controls blood pressure	Combats cancer	Strengthens the bones	Protects the heart	Aids in weight loss
Blueberries	Combats cancer	Protects the heart	Stabilizes blood sugar	Boosts memory	Prevents constipation
Broccoli	Strengthens the bones	Saves eye sight	Combats cancer	Protects the heart	Controls blood pressure
Cabbage	Combats cancer	Prevents constipation	Promotes weight loss	Protects the heart	Helps hemorrhoids
Cantaloupe	Saves the eye sight	Controls blood pressure	Lowers cholesterol	Combats cancer	Supports the immune system
Carrots	Saves the eye sight	Protects the heart	Prevents constipation	Combats cancer	Promotes weight loss
Cauliflower	Protects against prostate cancer	Combats breast cancer	Strengthens the bones	Banishes bruises	Guards against heart disease
Cherries	Protects the heart	Combats cancer	Ends insomnia	Slows the aging process	Shields against Alzheimer's
Chestnuts	Promotes weight loss	Protects the heart	Lowers cholesterol	Combats cancer	Controls blood pressure

Chili pepper	Aids digestion	Soothes sore throat	Combats cancer	Clears the sinuses	Boost the immune system
Figs	Promotes weight loss	Helps stop strokes	Lowers cholesterol	Combats cancer	Controls blood pressure
Fish	Protects the heart	Boosts memory	Protects the heart	Combats cancer	Supports the immune system
Flax	Aids in digestion	Battles diabetes	Protects the heart	Improves mental health	Boosts the immune system
Garlic	Lowers cholesterol	Controls blood pressure	Combats cancer	Kills bacteria	Fights fungus
Grapefruit	Protects against heart attacks	Promotes weight loss	Helps stop strokes	Combats prostate cancer	Lowers cholesterol
Grapes	Saves eye sight	Conquers kidney stones	Combats cancer	Enhances blood flow	Protects the heart
Green tea	Combats cancer	Protects the heart	Helps stop strokes	Promotes weight loss	Kills bacteria
Honey	Heals wounds	Aids in digestion	Guards against ulcers	Increase energy	Fights allergies
Lemons	Combats cancer	Protects the heart	Combats blood pressure	Smooths the skin	Stops scurvy
Limes	Combats cancer	Protects the heart	Controls blood pressure	Smooths the skin	Stops scurvy
Mangos	Combats cancer	Boosts memory	Regulates thyroid	Aids in digestion	Shields against Alzheimer's
Mushrooms	Controls blood pressure	Lowers cholesterol	Kills bacteria	Combats cancer	Strengthens the bones
Oats	Lowers cholesterol	Combats cancer	Battles diabetes	Prevents constipation	Smooths the skin
Olive oil	Protects the heart	Combats cancer	Promotes weight loss	Battles diabetes	Smooths the skin
Onions	Reduces risk of a heart attack	Combats cancer	Kills bacteria	Lowers cholesterol	Fights fungus
Oranges	Supports the immune system	Combats cancer	Protects the heart	Strengthens respirations	
Peaches	Prevents constipation	Combats cancer	Helps stop strokes	Aids in digestion	Helps hemorrhoids
Peanuts	Protects against heart disease	Promotes weight loss	Combats prostate cancer	Lowers cholesterol	Aggravates diverticulitis
Pineapple	Strengthens bones	Relieves colds	Aids in digestion	Dissolves warts	Blocks diarrhea
Prunes	Slows the aging process	Prevents constipation	Lowers cholesterol	Boosts memory	Protects against heart disease

Rice	Protects the heart	Battles diabetes	Conquers kidney stones	Combats cancer	Helps to stop strokes
Strawberries	Combats cancer	Protects the heart	Boosts memory	Calms stress	
Sweet potatoes	Saves the eye sight	Lifts mood	Combats cancer	Strengthens bones	
Tomatoes	Protects prostate	Combats cancer	Lowers cholesterol	Protects the heart	

declines, so says, Katherine Tucker, RD, PhD and chairperson of the department of health at the Northeastern University in Boston. Having this knowledge and knowing that there may be a decline in the body's ability to absorb certain nutrients completely with our food and the slowness of metabolizing it in our body due to the age process, these essential elements have become of increasing concern for our health and identification of and the use of these nutritional supplements have become important. Realizing that as it comes to human nutrition, we are still on a learning curve about nutrition but what we do know are some important facts regarding key nutrients that we notice are in short supply in the human body as we age. Please understand that eating a variety of foods is the best way to get the nutrients you need but for most of us, I do not see this happening because of our lifestyle. Your doctor may even recommend a supplement that is deficient in your diet. Here are some of the supplements that may be of benefit. I have taken the liberty of identifying the foods in greater detail because other supplements will have the same foods nutrients as above and you can refer to these listed nutrients for clarity and better understanding. These supplements are in no order of importance because they are all important. The **recommended daily intake (RDI)** will be given if known.

Vitamin B12 (Cobalamin)

The body cannot make B12 and it is one of the powerhouses of the vitamin world. It is part of the DNA, the nervous system and of the blood cells. B12 is an essential and extremely important vitamin for the health of the brain as well as our immune system. The hormones, actually, the entire body's metabolism could not run smoothly without this essential vitamin. The recommended daily intake of B12 is 2.4mcg daily but slightly higher in pregnant and nursing mothers. It is called an intrinsic vitamin which means that it is absorbed by the stomach with the help of proteins. Proteins bind to the B12 molecule to help it absorb into the blood stream to the cells. This is one vitamin that can be stored in the liver for later use. B12 is mainly an animal and dairy product vitamin but there are many foods that have been fortified with this vitamin. Plants that contain natural sources of vitamin B12 include dried and fermented plants such as tempeh, nori, and laver (a seaweed). There are other algae rich in B12 such as Porphyra yezoensis a seaweed that contain the same amount of B12 as the liver. Foods that have a high percentage of B12 are:

Fish contain vitamin B12 such as salmon, trout, tuna, sardines, and clams to mention a few. Most fish are also high in Omega 3, proteins, phosphorus, selenium and some have zinc, manganese, iron, and other B vitamins.

Fortified food such as non-dairy milk, nutritional yeast, and fortified cereals. Read the label package to determine other fortified supplements in the food.

Whole milk and milk products such as yogurt and cheese are high in B12 and proteins. **Eggs** are a great source of B12, B2, and proteins. The egg yolk has the highest amount of B12 compared to the egg white.

Beef, animal liver, and kidneys are excellent sources of B12 as well as B2, B3, and B6, selenium, and zinc. This concept of not eating meat is not totally correct. In many ways lean meat is the only true way of obtaining the nutrients necessary in the qualities, and quantities required for biological health. Choose low fat cuts of meat for a higher concentration of B12. Liver and kidneys have the most nutrients and lamb are the richest in B12, B2, selenium, and proteins.

Vitamin B6 (Pyridoxine)

Vitamin B6 is important for the normal brain development and for keeping the nervous system and immune system health. Food sources are poultry, fish, potatoes, chickpeas, and bananas. The RBI is 1.5mg to 1.7mg daily.

Vitamin D2, D3, (Calciferol)

Vitamin D is a group of five vitamins that are fat-soluble secosteriods (a form of steroid) that is responsible for increasing the absorption in the intestinal track of calcium, magnesium, and phosphate. Vitamin D has a number of other biological effects in humans. There are a group of vitamin D's but the most important are **D3 or cholecalciferol** and **D2 or ergocalciferol.** Vitamin D3 comes from sun exposure more specifically UVB radiation and yes D3 and D2 can be ingested from a diet or from supplements. Many foods and fluids are fortified with vitamin D. Once ingested into the body and the diet, vitamin D has to be converted through a process of hydroxylation to convert it to an active form. This conversion is done in the liver and kidney. Vitamin D is not technically a vitamin. It is more of a hormone or sterol/steroid. The RDI dose is from 600IU (International Units) to not more than 4,000IU daily.

Vitamin B3 (Niacinamide or Nicotinic acid)

Vitamin B3 or niacin is a water-soluble vitamin and is not stored in the body. There are two forms of these vitamins: **Nicotinic acid** is the form used to lower cholesterol, the other form is **Niacinamide or** nicotinamide and does not lower cholesterol but it may help treat psoriasis and reduce risk of non-melanoma skin cancer. Niacin (nicotinic acid) is an important nutrient that is in every part of your body. To mention a few of the benefits, this vitamin may help in reducing cholesterol, ease arthritis, and increase brain function, and help with pellagra. Through the foods that is ingested, the body can make niacin in small amounts as long as it has the amino acid tryptophan. Some of the food sources are tuna, salmon, turkey, pork, veal, spices such as sesame seeds, ginger, sweet peppers, portobello mushrooms, sunflower seeds, and some vegetables. It is also in fortified foods. RDI recommended daily dose is 500mg to 1000mg.

Vitamin B9 (Folate or Folic acid)

Vitamin B9 is a water-soluble vitamin. Folate is the natural form that occurs naturally in nature in many foods and is acquired from the diet which makes it an essential vitamin. Folic acid is the manufacture brand of folate which convert to folate in the body once ingested. The RDI (recommended daily intake) of folate or folic acid is 400mcg from dietary supplements. In some countries this is a fortified vitamin in certain foods. Folate is especially important during periods of frequent cell division and growth, such as, infancy and pregnancy. This vitamin is important for DNA's continuous cell division and RNA transcription and subsequent protein synthesis. Sources of Vitamin B9 are beans, lentils, spinach, asparagus, lettuce, avocado, broccoli, oranges, whole wheat bread. RDI recommended daily dose is 400mcg to 1,000mcg.

Vitamin E (Tocopherol)

Vitamin E is a group of 8 fat-soluble compounds that include four tocopherols and four tocotrienols. Vitamin E helps to maintain healthy cells and poor vision, gout, cardiovascular disease, and possibly dementia, cancer, and also arthritis. It is an antioxidant which means it helps to slow down the aging process of damaged cells. Vitamin E is found in plants and animal foods but the best source of tocopherols is found in plants such as vegetables, seeds, and nut oils. The oil component of all grains contains Vitamin E and most of this is lost in the milling or refinement of the grain. If you are taking medication, your doctor should be advised that you are taking Vitamin E. Vitamin E can decrease the beneficial effects of some vitamins such as niacin, beta-carotene, and vitamin C. Tocopherols Vitamin E can be found in butter, egg yolks, milk fat, and in the liver. RDI recommended amount is 400IU daily.

Calcium

Calcium is a mineral and is the most neglected nutrient in the elder populations' diet yet it is the most important mineral for the building and maintenance of a strong bone structure. Calcium works with Vitamin D and other minerals to keep the bones strong for all age groups. If this mineral is not taken in by ingestion, the body will siphon or take the calcium from the bones and teeth to satisfy the needs of the rest of the body. This will increase the risk of **osteoporosis** and other bone dyscrasias and may possible contribute to fractures. Calcium can be found in milk and milk products, canned fish with soft bone, dark green leafy vegetables, oranges juice with fortified calcium, as well as fortified cereals. The RDI is 1,000mg to not more then 2,000mg.

Potassium

Potassium is an important mineral for cellular and electrolyte functions in the body. It is the most abundant intracellular cation (electrolyte) within all tissues because it is required to maintain the fluid volume and balance within the cells. Potassium has a strong relationship with sodium which regulates extracellular (fluid volume outside the cell), including plasma volume. Potassium can balance the negative effects of sodium (salt) with the reduction of sodium and can lower your blood pressure. Foods high in potassium are; spinach, broccoli, potatoes, mushrooms, peas, cucumbers, and others. RDI recommendations of daily intake is 2,600 mg to 3,400mg

Fiber (Roughage)

Fiber is a part of the plant that cannot be completely broken down or digested by human enzymes. There are two main types: **Soluble fiber** which can dissolve in water and is readily fermented in the colon and can extend the feeling of fullness – **Insoluble fiber** do not dissolve in water and is not digested by enzymes in the upper gastrointestinal track. It does absorb water as it moves through the digestive system easing defecation. The health benefits of dietary fiber and whole grains may include a decrease risk of death and lower rate of coronary heart disease, colon cancer, and type 2 diabetes.

Acetyl-L-Carnitine (ALCAR)

ALCAR is a **mitochondrial** boosting supplement that improves mood, learning, and memory. ALCAR will help your muscles mitochondria burn fat which can increase endurance, give you more energy for activities and an added edge in the gym, helps in blood glucose regulation, and it will help you to recover faster. Foods with ALCAR are mainly animal products, dairy, poultry, and meats. Red meats have the highest concentration. There is no RDI of ALCAR but 3g daily is a good dose.

Omega-3 fatty acids

Omega-3 cannot be produced in the body on its own, you must get this nutrient from your diet. There are three important types: ALA (alpha-linolenic acid), DHA (docosahexaenoic acid), and EPA (eicosapentaenoic acid). ALA is found in plants and DHA and EPA is found in animal foods and algae. As your brain ages the brain cells gradually lose the ability to absorb DHA, starving the mind and compromising the brain and memory of its retention abilities. Omega-3 studies have linked brain benefits ranging from better blood flow and increase growth of brain cells and increase in mood enhancement to Omega. Omega-3 helps prevent irregular heartbeats, reduce plaque buildup in the arteries, inhibit inflammation, and keep the blood sugar level in check. RDI recommended daily intake is 1000mg of EPA and DHA of Omega-3 daily. Good source Flaxseed oil, salmon, walnuts, edamame (immature soybeans).

Herbal Supplements

Herbal supplements are the use of plants or parts of the plants like the root, leaves, and wood for medicinal purposes and as you can see all parts of the plant are used. This science is called herbology or herbalism and is the true study of botany. When we talk about herbal supplement, we are talking about supplements that come from different parts of the plant and some of the herbal supplement's names will be familiar to you such as gingko biloba, ginseng, echinacea, St. John's wort, aloe, licorice root, kava- kava, ginger, garlic, and black cohosh. Plants have been used as medicine for much of the human evolution and are still studied and practiced to this day. Evidence of herbal use was found that dates back to the **Paleolithic** age almost 60,000 years ago. Herbal remedies date back to the Sumerians, Egyptians, Babylonians,

Indians, Native Americans, Chinese, and Greeks. They were all herbalists to some extent with some of the written medicinal practices dating back as long as 5,000 years ago. One of the oldest written use of herbs for medicinal purposes was on papyruses found in Egypt. It is the lengthiest writings on herbal use ever discovered and covering over 700 herbal drugs from plant origin. It was called the **Ebers Papyrus** and dates back to 1550 BC. The Greek herbals writings came from **Theophrastus of Eresos** which dates back to the 4th c. BC. Ancient India used herbs as a primary treatment for disease. Since the Bronze Age c.1600-c1046 BC, in ancient China during the Shang Dynasty sketches and seeds were found describing use of the seeds as herbal medicine. In the **Huang Neijing** over 224 drugs are mentioned in the text were herbs. The **World Health Organization (WHO)** believes that at least 80 percent of Asia and Africa use herbal medicine as their primary health care source. I have to admit that I have used these herbal supplements myself and have found them to be of great help to me. It is true that herbology may be more psychological than actual but even that is something positive. Many of our present medicines are derived from the essence of herbal harvesting. Those that are not are manipulations and/or synthesis of the actual herb.

Safety and Effectiveness of Herbal Supplements

Studies have been conducted at a number of health departments to determine if herbal therapy were suitable for coverage by health insurance companies but as of this time no clear evidence can be found for the effectiveness, use, and medical value for coverage. In 2010, there was a survey of 1000 herbs plant-derivatives and only 156 of these had clinical trials. There was strong evidence that some (5) were toxic and allergic and nine plants had some evidence of therapeutic effect. There was no known evidence that any herbal remedy can treat cancer. If you are using modern pharmaceutical medicine and herbal medicine you should check with your physician. Plant herbs and pharmaceutical drugs can interact causing very serious adverse effects that may be dangerous to your health.

After all of this, it would seem that herbs would be safe since some herbs are used all the time when we cook. These are the safer ones. This may not be the case for some other herbs.

St. John's wort is sometimes used for depression, anxiety, and to help one to sleep better but it can cause side effects such as dizziness, nausea, dry mouth, and headaches. It also attracts UVR or the sunlight so you are more likely to get a sunburn. As with all supplements, your doctor should be told if you are taking this herb.

Kava-kava is used to help with insomnia and anxiety but you should not take it if you have liver or kidney problems. Alcohol, as with most other medications, should not be taken with kava-kava because it may cause sleepiness.

Ginkgo biloba is often taken to improve memory, increase circulation, increase mental functioning, and can alleviate altitudes sickness as well as other conditions. What is not known about ginkgo is that it can thin your blood and if you are taking any blood thinning medications, it is wise to avoid this herb.

Ginger is used to relieve and ease nausea especially with women during pregnancy and menstruation. It is used as an autoinflammatory, as a relaxant for the stomach after chemotherapy, to prevent or control motion sickness, to improve respiratory problems, and some have used it for arthritis and joint pain. Side effects are heartburn, diarrhea, and general stomach discomfort.

Aloe is good for wounds and burns and will help in the healing process. The healing will be faster and it would make the wounds feel better. There are those that have taken Aloe by mouth and in some cases, this can cause abnormal stomach discomfort and heart rhythm complications or kidney problems. It may also lower your blood sugar level if you have diabetes.

Ginseng is a group of herbs that is known as an energy booster and some take it because it is said to help in slowing down the aging process. It is also taken as a booster in increasing immunity or to help with sex functions. Do not take it if you are taking any blood thinners or if you have pre-or pro diabetes or have a fluctuation in glucose levels.

Black cohosh is a supplement often used for menopause symptoms like hot flashes and night sweats. It can also be used to help with premenstrual syndrome (PMS). It should be avoided by those with liver problems and breast cancer.

Garlic is used to help lower high blood pressure and to treat cold symptoms. It has been studied and shown to lower your cholesterol levels. Garlic can thin your blood and increase your risk of bleeding if you are on blood thinning medications.

Licorice root is used to treat coughs, stomach ulcers, bronchitis, infections, and sore throats. Licorice has been known to raise your blood pressure, cause heart rhythms problems, and can exacerbate or precipitate problems with the kidney.

Echinacea is used to fight the flu, help to control blood sugar, aids in the growth of cells, helps manages anxiety, and has been known to lower inflammation. Echinacea does have an effect on the immune system and can increase the white blood cells. The most common side effect is upset stomach and worsening asthma symptoms,

A Little More on Antioxidants and the Older Adults

Although we have covered this earlier, this is a good chapter to give a little more information on antioxidants. Oxidation is a chemical reaction that involves the removing of an electron and it is the substances that gives away the electron that has been oxidized. Example: It is similar to the process of iron rusting (oxidization). As the cells are broken down by free-radicals or other means of oxidization, antioxidants slow down this process and protect the cells from damage and dying. There many good antioxidants and I will name just a few:

Allium sulphur compound – leeks, onions, and garlic
Beta-carotene – carrots, spinach, pumpkin, and mangos
Copper – seafood, lean meat, milk, and nuts
Catechins – red wine and tea
Flavonoids – tea, green tea, citrus fruits, red wine, onions, and apples
Lycopene – tomatoes, pink grapefruit, and watermelon
Luteins – green leafy vegetables like spinach, and corn
Manganese – seafood, lean meat, milk, and nuts
Selenium – seafood, lean meat, and whole grain
Vitamin C – oranges, mangos, kiwi, broccoli, and strawberries
Vitamin E – vegetable oil (such as wheatgerm), avocados, seeds, whole grains, & nuts

Antioxidants as in herbal supplements in large amounts and in large concentrations can be harmful and may increase oxidation. It could actually protect and/or harm the cells if used in large amounts which will reduce the health benefits of exercise and actually cause side effects and even reach toxic levels. Everything in moderation and if you are thinking about using supplements study them and learn as much about them as you can. See if they fit into your health needs then talk to your doctor, pharmacies, and/or registered dietitian. What works for some may not work for you, check the websites for information. Please be aware, just because something is said to be all natural does not mean that it is safe. If you're taking any medications even those that are over-the-counter (OTC) like allergy medications, weight control pills, aspirins or even Tylenol this also includes vitamins, minerals, and herbs your doctor needs to know what these supplements are and the frequency you are taking them. Enclosed is an herbal chart on traditional Chinese herbal remedies with treatments as well as a more domestic herbal chart that I think you may find interesting. Buy wisely, use responsibly, and be knowledgeable about all health supplements.

Nutritional foods/Supplements for the Elder at a Glance

Nutritional Supplements	RDI/ Amounts Needed	Purpose of Supplement	Food Source of Nutrient
Vitamin B12 (Cobalamin group)	2.4 mcg daily	Vitamin B12 is a group of cobalamins that are water soluble vitamins. The body cannot make B12 so it needs a daily intake supple of B12. It is essential for the DNA, nervous system, immune system, and the blood.	Vitamin B12 is mainly an animal and dairy product vitamin but there are many foods that have been fortified with B12. Most fish products, Salmon, clams, tuna etc.
Vitamin D (Calciferol group)	600 IU daily to not more than 4,000 IU daily	Vitamin D is a group of fat-soluble secosteriods or hormones called vitamins that helps in increasing the absorption in the intestinal tract of calcium, magnesium, B 12, and phosphorus with many other biological effects.	Vitamin D comes from UVB radiation (sun) and is fortified in foods. Foods that contain Vitamin D are fatty fish like salmon, tuna, mackerel and fish liver oil. Small amounts are in meat, livers, cheese, and egg yolk. Milk products are fortified with Vit. D.
Vitamin B6 (Pyridoxine)	1.5 mg to 1.7 mg daily	Vitamin B6 is a water-soluble vitamin that helps the body maintain normal brain development keeping the nervous system and the immune system healthy.	Vitamin B3 good sources are poultry, most fish, potatoes, chickpeas and bananas.
Vitamin B3 (Niacin)	500mg to 1,000 mg daily	Vitamin B3 is a water-soluble vitamin that is not stored in the body. There are two forms of this vitamin one can lower cholesterol the other can help treat psoriasis and reduce non-melanoma skin cancer. Both can ease arthritis, and increase brain function.	Vitamin B3 can be found in tuna, salmon, turkey. pork, veal, venison, veal, and spices. Some of the spices are sesame seeds, ginger, sweet pepper, sunflower seeds, portobello mush-room, and some vegetables.
Vitamin B9 (Folate or folic acid)	400 mcg to 100mcg daily	Vitamin B9 is important for the continuation of cell DNA division and function especially during pregnancy and infancy growth. It is important for RNA transcription and protein synthesis. It is also used for anemia.	Vitamin B9 can be found in beans, lentils, spinach, asparagus, lettuce, avocado, broccoli, oranges, and whole wheat bread.

Vitamin E (Tocopherol group)	400 IU daily	Vitamin E is a group of tocopherols that maintains healthy cells, helps poor vision, prevents gout, can be used to help cardiovascular disease, and may be good for dementia, cancer and arthritis. It is an antioxidant and can help slow down the aging process in cells.	Vitamin E is found in plants and animals alike but the best source is found in plants such as most vegetables, seeds and nut oil. The oil component of all grains contains tocopherols. It also can be found in butter, egg yolk, milk fat, and in liver.
Calcium	1,000 mg to 2,000 mg daily	Calcium is a mineral that is important to build strong bones and teeth. Calcium works with Vit. D and other minerals to keep the bones and teeth strong for all ages but is especially important for females after menopause. Low calcium intake will increase the risk of osteoporosis or other bone dyscrasias.	Calcium can be found in milk and milk products, canned fish with soft bones, dark green leafy vegetables, orange juice that is fortified, and calcium fortified cereals.
Fiber (Soluble and Insoluble)	25 g to 38 g daily	Fiber is from plants and cannot be broken down or ingested. There 3 types of soluble and insoluble forms. They produce the bulk, viciousness, and fermentation in the intestinal tract and this regulates the fecal elimination.	Fibers are from plant foods and come from cereal, fruits, vegetables, wheat, barley, legumes, soybeans, and peas as well as many other plant foods.
Potassium	2,600 mg to 3,400 mg daily	Potassium is a mineral for cellular and electrical functions in the body and is the most abundant electrolyte. It maintains the fluid volume and balance. Potassium has a strong relationship with sodium that regulates fluid volume outside and inside the cells and both control your blood pressure.	Potassium can be found in spinach, broccoli, potatoes, mushrooms, peas, cucumbers, coconuts, all nuts, yams, milk, chocolate, bananas, and parsley.
Acetyl-L-Carnitine (ALCAR)	250 mg to 500 mg	ALCAR is a mitochondrial booster nutrient that is the most abundant in the body. It is stated that it helps muscle burn fat which will increase endurance, increase energy, and help one recover faster.	ALCAR can be found in animal products, dairy products, poultry, and meats. Red meats have the highest concentration of ALCAR.
Omega-3 (Fatty acid group)	1,000 mg	Omega-3 is regarded as an essential fatty acid and is a group of fatty acids that are not produced in the body and must be ingested. ALA is found in plants and EPA and DHA are found in animals and also algae. Omega-3 helps cell growth, increases blood flow, and enhanced one's mood. It also helps to reduce plaque build-up in the arteries.	Omega-3 can be found in flaxseed oil, salmon, walnuts

Herbals Supplements at a Glance

Herbal Supplement	Benefits Side Effects
Aloe	Good for wounds and burns and will help to heal them faster and make them feel better. There are those that have taken Aloe by mouth and in some cases, this can cause abnormal stomach discomfort and heart rhythm complications or kidney problems. It may also lower your blood sugar levels if you have diabetes.
Black cohosh	This supplement is often used for menopause symptoms like hot flashes and night sweats, and also can be used to help with PMS. It should be avoided by those with liver problems and breast cancer.
Echinacea	Used to fight the flu, help to control blood sugar, aids in the growth of cells, helps manages anxiety, and has been known to lower inflammation. Echinacea does have an effect on the immune system and can increase the white blood cells. The most common side effect is upset stomach and worsening asthma symptoms,
Garlic	Is used to help lower high blood pressure and to treat cold symptoms. It has been researched and studied that it can lower your cholesterol levels. Garlic can thin your blood and increase your risk of bleeding if you are on blood thinning medications.
Ginger	Used to relieve and ease nausea especially with women during pregnancy and menstruation, used as an anti-inflammatory, as a relaxant for the stomach after chemotherapy, to prevent or control motion sickness, used to improve respiratory problems, and some have used it for arthritis and joint pain. Side effects are heartburn, diarrhea, and general stomach discomfort.
Ginkgo biloba	Often taking to improve memory, increase circulation, increase mental functioning, and can alleviate altitudes sickness as well as other conditions. What is also known about ginkgo is that it can thin your blood and if you are taking any blood thinning medications, it is wise to avoid this herb.
Ginseng	A group of herbs that is known as an energy booster. It has been used to help in slowing down the aging process. It is also taken as a booster in helping to increase immunity or to help with all sexual functions. Do not take it if you are taking any blood thinners or if you are pre-or pro to diabetes or have a fluctuation in glucose levels.
Kava-kava	Suppose to help with insomnia and anxiety but you should not take it if you have liver or kidney problems. Alcohol and other medications with kava-kava do not mix and may cause sleepiness.
Licorice root	Is used to treat coughs, stomach ulcers, bronchitis, infections, and sore throats. Licorice has been known to raise your blood pressure, cause heart rhythm problems, and can exacerbate or precipitate a problem with the kidney.
St. John's wort	Sometimes used for depression, anxiety, and to help one to sleep better but it can cause side effects such as dizziness, nausea, dry mouth, and headaches. It also attracts UVR or sunlight so you are more likely to get a sunburn. As with all supplements, your doctor should be told if you are taking this or any nutritional supplements.

Traditional Chinese Herbal Supplements at a Glance

Superior Tonic Herb Chart

Traditional Chinese Medicine (TCM) believe that all health challenges are caused by imbalances. "Excesses" occur when too much heat, cold dampness, dryness, phlegm, toxins, or stagnation. "Deficiencies" stem from the lack of vital energy Qi (Vital), Jing (Essence), or Stem (Mind). Abundant health is considered possible only when the body is in perfect balance.

Herbs	Benefits	Lungs	Spleen	Liver	Kidney	Heart	Blood	Sing	Qi	Chen
		Organ Systems						Treasures		
American Ginseng (Panax Quinquefolium Xi Yang Stem)	American Ginseng differs from Panax Ginseng in that it is cooling rather than warming. Good for those with heart conditions, smokers, and those living in smoggy areas. Noted for its ability to promote the secretion of bodily fluids. Helps to moisten the lungs. Great energy tonic for those in hot climates.	X	X					X	X	X
Asparagus Root (Tan Men Dong)	Asparagus Root is widely used to maintain beautiful skin, increase vitality, and establish a happy outlook on life. It is thought to help balance the entire body. Good lung tonic for those that smoke, live in desert climates or are regularly exposed to smog. Helps lungs extract oxygen from the air we breathe, and helps remove toxins from the lungs.	X		X	X			X	X	X
Astragalus Root (Huang Qi)	Astragalus Root is believed to strengthen the primary energy of the body and improve all metabolic functions. Special benefit to the respiratory and elimination system. Known as a potent physiological energizer and for helping to benefit muscle tone. Extremely important in helping the skin eliminate toxins.	X	X						X	
Codonopsis Root (Dang Shen)	Codonopsis Root is among the most widely used of all Superior Tonic Herbs. It is extremely mild, presents no side-effects, but is among the premiere Qi tonic. Blood building agency for those weakened by illness. Promotes function of both the spleen and the lung systems. Enhances interferon production. Blood and immune tonic.	X	X			X			X	

Cordyceps (Dong Chong Xia)	Cordyceps replenishes the energy loss to excessive exertion, stress, illness, injury or aging. A kidney tonic that supports sexual function, brain power, skeletal integrity, and healing ability. Widely used to overcome back aches. Potent lung tonic beneficial for those who require strong respiratory from exercise or injury. Shown to help resist a large range of pathogenic fungi, viruses and bacteria.	X			X			X	X	
Dong Quai (Angelica Sinensis)	Dong Quai is a blood tonic that treat anemia and can help rebuild red blood cells after illness, injuries, or surgery. It helps increase the volume of blood. TCM's most universal gynecological herb, and is used in formulas to treat painful or lack of menstruation, premenstrual syndrome, infertility, and menopause distress. Helpful for skin blemishes, urticaria, eczema, neuro-dermatitis.		X	X			X			
Eleuthero Root (Siberian Ginseng Acanthopanax)	Eleuthero Root is a tremendous adaptogen and is known as a premiere tonic for the adrenal glands. It increases physical strength, sharpens concentration, increases visual ability, and healing powers. Promotes lean body weight and both long and short term energy. Widely used to prevent altitude sickness and minimizes stress damage.	X	X	X	X	X		X	X	
Epimedium (Yin Tang Huo)	Epimedium is considered to be the most powerful aphrodisiac herb derived from plant source. It is very famous for its power to strengthening sexual power in men, and in some cases women. It is thought to be strengthening to the body as a whole, it is remarkably rejuvenating and its invigorating effect is legendary in China. Epimedium is known as "Passionate Goat Herb" in China for increasing the sexual desires and increasing sperm production as well as stimulating sensory nerves.			X	X			X	X	
Eucommia Bark (Du Zhong)	Eucommia Bark is remarkably potent for building a strong and flexible skeletal. It is also good for strengthening the bones, ligaments, and tendons. It is among the finest of all kidney tonics for function. It is a mild diuretic and anti-inflammatory and can ease the systems of high blood pressure.			X	X			X		

Chapter 9

The Art of Exertion

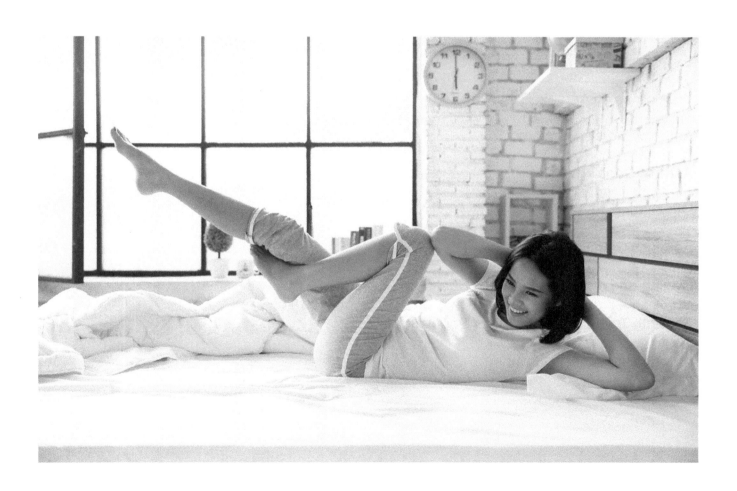

Contents in Chapter 9

The Art of Exertion

Being a very active person and raised in a number of institutions where the atmosphere was heavy into sports activities the propensity of the day was to better the other students in your unit in any and all forms of sports activities so it is hard to image not being hyperactive in some form when it comes to any challenging events. Exercising was like a drug and a challenge was the overdose of that drug in which action had to be made. This attitude is what carried me throughout most of my life but one starts to learn that this perception is not the norm; in fact, it is the opposite of the socially acceptable normal psyche of the time. Most of the population are not this energetic and do not have or pose this type of challenging mode of conduct. Again, this was my norm or the same type of modus operandi as when I grew up and learned to expect life's behavior to be and/or appreciated. I dear say that I have learned that active individuals perform their most active activities at their regular day to day jobs. Some of these jobs are as active as any actual exercise program one can participate in but are in many different job settings; nurses are constantly on their feet taking care of patients, building porters and superintendents of buildings are constantly pulling, lifting and dragging things in and out of their buildings, firemen are running up and down burning buildings with heavy loads on their backs and shoulders rescuing tenants, sanitation workers are constantly lifting heavy bags, furniture and heaving these loads into their trucks, police officers are constantly on their feet walking their beat, postal workers are walking their postal routes delivering mail, and so-on-and-so-forth to mention a few of the many other hard working people doing very active and strenuous jobs on a daily bases. One begins to wonder if this exertion is the same thing as doing exercise? If not, then what do we mean when we use the word "exercise."

Brief History of Exertion

It is said that exercise physiology actually started in Asia Minor and Greece but in reality, it started even earlier than that, it started at the very dawn of civilization the beginning of mankind. Physical strength was a necessary survival skill and being physically fit was a prime requisite for survival requirement. This struggle for existence was the difference in being able to make it through this day to see the next day and the next and this continued for all living things for many millenniums. Survival skills was also the mode and means to find out who will be the dominant specie on this planet earth and the homo sapiens evidentially prevailed. It was not just because of their physical prowess that propelled and helped them through, but as this species longevity continued its survival extension, motor skills and dexterity developed as well as, and most importantly, the growth of their information gathering skills developed as the homo sapiens brain continued to grow and absorb its surroundings and use it for dominance. As homo sapiens continued to evolve and their brains continued absorbing more and more knowledge and understanding about their environment; their physical form and their abilities to use this form and new information to learn to grasp objects, balance on two feet, and find shelter all became a means of protection for these wandering nomads. This evolution slowly but assuredly improved for the homo sapiens as they continued developing new skills and progressiveness of endurances in all fields due to the continuous enlargement of their brain. The next stage is to form gangs or groups for added defense and protection. Societal gangs or packs were ultimately formed for added protection and this ultimately brought about the distribution of work responsibilities, to support these gathering packs or groups and new roles within the groups developed, leaders developed or were chosen leading eventually to an actual social gathering and then to an ordered community. This happened in many different continents and at different times but within these gatherings, rules of living arose and law and order were formed. As mankind continued to mature in these many different continents with different forms of socialization, so did different stages of civilization that were required, growth in cultural and advancement in knowledge and also progression in societal skills. Human development became more organized in their thinking, needs, and the onset of sociability to meet the growing populations society formed; enlightenment prevailed in many continents. Mankind developed their own cultural identities, cities grew and governments were shaped some flourished others did not, different structures of law and order was introduced, religious beliefs grew, and social values were nurtured.

Health practices also thrived throughout the known civilized world especially in Asia Minor and Greece. In Greece, during the 5th century (500-401 BC), a Greek physician and philosopher Herodicus, believed that actively working out and hard physical training is a therapeutic treatment for keeping and maintaining good health and in the prevention of diseases. He promulgated that hard-exertive training coupled with a good diet, massage, herbs, and oils is the key to the maintenance of health. Herodicus, who was an athlete himself, theorized that sports training and the addition of proper living as stated above are considered to be the foundation for good health and a longer life. Herodicus is considered to be the father of sports medicine. Another great Greek physician Claudius Galen – (129-199/217 AD), a follower of Herodicus as well as of Hippocrates and a supporter of their medical principals also postulated that diet, fitness, and good health measures will enhance life. In one of Galen's books called **"The Laws of Health"** he wrote as followed **"Breathe fresh air, eat proper foods, drink the right beverages, hard physical training, get adequate sleep, have a daily bowel movement, and control emotions."** Does this sound familiar to you? He felt that this was the key to good health and longevity. The beginning of physical training and the health benefits it imparts has a long and lustrous history. The concern for keeping and maintaining good health in the attempt to thwart off diseases is still with us today and even during the earliest part of man's long survival mode it still is part of our everyday practice and will be in the future. From ancient civilization to present it has become the greatest impact to the Western civilization and to the rest of the world the fact that hard physical training and good nutrition are the key to a healthy and long-lasting life. This is all well and good but it still does not answer the question as to what is meant by the word

exercise so I went into Wikipedia for an answer and all they can say about exercise is that it is **"any bodily activity that enhances or maintains physical fitness and overall health and wellness."** Then it goes on to give a whole scenario as to why it is performed and the reasons for its use. Again, this is all well and good but it does not answer the question "is very hard and strenuous work such as a job like farming equal to or conceded to be a form of exercise." Looking to other sources I found out that the first recorded use of the actual word exercise came from England in the late 14th century. The meaning of the word exercise at that time was "condition of being in active operation; practice for the sake of training" and in France it means "execution of power; physical or spiritual exercise?"

Jerry Morris, MD and Epidemiologist, was born in Liverpool and raised in Glasgow (May 06, 1910 – October 28, 2009) has been credited for putting together a more scientific correlations of being physically active and using the association of exertion with cardiovascular disease and heart disease, he came up with a theory. He wrote in his inspiring paper that there is a link between exercise and the reduction in cardiovascular and heart disease. He was the first to physiologically associate physical training or exertion and a specific disease, "Heart Disease." Jerry Morris, MD is considered "the man who invented exercises for the prevention of heart disease." I can go on and on from the ancient Chinese and to India's physical training and health endeavors and their strive in the prevention of diseases and increasing longevity, to their therapeutic movements and stretching techniques but there you have it. I can write about all of their health benefits that came from Yoga, massage therapy, herbology, meditation, and make this treatise as a history lesson and name ancient, modern, and present exercise physiologist but that is not what this text is about. It is enough to say that physical training and all that was just mentioned was promulgated in the hope and benefits of ensuring good health and in living a longer life. Hard work is a form of exercise and does fall under the meaning "being in active operation" or "the execution of power" as the original of the word were intended to be. Albeit, is this what we mean this day and age as to the meaning of exercise? I think not. Exercise to me means **"performing activities above what is considered a person's normal daily active."** Being a fireman or a farmer, a nurse or working in construction as an everyday job is strenuous work, this is absolutely correct, but it is **your** "normal daily everyday activity" and normal daily activities are different and should be separated from physical training or exercise modalities. **Planned exercise or physical training is different and is a job unto itself** but it is a very principled, repetitive, tenuous, and a conditioning type of a job for the body, mind, and spirit. **This is your alone time your personal time.** The one time out of a hard day at work that you have found for yourself to work on you and your health. It should be a sacred time where you challenge and discipline your body and your mind to perform to the best of its ability, to achieve inner wholeness and spiritual guidance, and to balance life's internal and external stresses. **Your Yin/Yang Time.**

What is Exercise?

No matter where you look for the meaning of "exercise" you will find a different interpretation, meaning or concept as to this word. For us older folks, when the doctor tells us to 'do more exercise' it is hard to put that into a picture or to understand what exercise he wants us to do.

The doctor does not give us an exercise algorithm list and we know what exercise means in a personal sense and in this context, we visualize the movement of increasing our drive to be more active. We also know that movement activities are meant to increase our heart rate, work our muscles, and eventually with this added activity hopefully be able to burn more calories. We get it. Albeit, what activities should we do, should we join a gym, hire a trainer, and most importantly how much will it cost. Making these suggestions sounds very professional and nice to the doctor but how do we go about do these things and how do we get started? There's no real answer to these questions although one idea is that you learn what it is your getting yourself into which is to learn the very basics of what the concept of exercise is. You have to decide what you need and how to go about doing the exertion/exercise. The question is why am I doing it? Is it just because the doctor told me to?

Introduction to Exercise

Before starting an endeavor of physical activities, it is important for one to find out why one would want to do this tedious extra work. If this is not settled in your mind then you will find many reasons to start-stop-start-stop or just start and stop. Nothing is easy and when it comes to exercise and physical activities nothing is fast, over night or tomorrow. It will take time, perseverance, and repetitiveness to see results. It is a common feeling for many exercise enthusiasts to find excuses not to take that walk around the block; stop the excuses and just do it. Putting in a hard-physical program before or after a long day of work is difficult and challenging but also very rewarding in its health benefits. It is the same with those of us that have retired and/or may be in need of added health assistance. Learning about physical fitness requires some understanding of what it means to be in a fit condition. That requires understanding of three basic principles – **Frequency, Intensity, Time (F.I.T.).** This follows what is part of the **Overload Principle** better known as **Specificity** and if tracked and done properly will provide regular imposed demands and stress or **S.A.I.D.** which means **specific adaption to imposed demands – See Glossary).** All exercises or fitness programs must have these stated concepts to work as their main training factors in any and all exercise programs: Read the book - Health and Physical Fitness: For the Beginner.

Frequency is how often you plan on doing a program of exercise or physical activities that is above your normal every day events. Are you going to exercise twice a week, three times a week or more? It can also mean repetitiveness of movement in the exercise.

Intensity depends on the amount of effort, force, strength, or energy as well as how much you feel about what you are doing (mental strength). It also has to do with the quality and quantity of the force or resistance or energy demands used.

Time you will allow yourself to complete your program of exercise: One hour, two hours, and so-on. This can also refer to the time between movement or between distance of each set or bout.

Exercise is a conglomeration of many activities thrust together with no beginning but a definite end: improvement. In physical activities, the basic categories or types of exercises that one can do for fitness fall under **cardiovascular system, muscle endurance, muscle strength, balance, flexibility, and body composition.** Each type of exercise mentioned is different in some way to the physiological outcome but are all beneficial in its result of producing force, strenuous effort, and energy production. All this is related to physical activities and are known as **exertion.** The majority of people tend to focus their attention on just one specific category or form of exertion but a program with an equal portion of all four is best. This is what is known as cross-training. Working all four activities into your exercise routine will effectively work most of the muscles in the body and will improve any sport you have chosen. In order to make exercise affective, F.I.T. is the main ingredient in degrees and demands that must be used in all four of these activities.

Cardiovascular or cardiorespiratory is the prolong ability of the heart and lungs to supply the muscles with nutrients and oxygen.

Muscle endurance is the ability of the muscles to exert activity for extended periods of time. It is used in aerobic and in some anaerobic activities that increases your heart and breathing rate.

Muscle strength can be described as the ability to contract your muscles to resist forces, pressure, and gravity. In exercise, it is the movement of contracting and relaxing your muscles repetitively to make them stronger: **Static strength** – how much weight you can hold or **Dynamic strength** – how much weight you can move.

Balance is the equal distribution of weight on all sides making it easier to walk on all surfaces which helps to prevent falls.

Flexibility commonly describes as **range of motion (ROM)** around a particular joint or set of joints. Basically, ROM means how far one can bend, reach or turn. Many associate ROM and flexibilities as stretching as the same thing but they are very different. **Stretching** is a form of exercise that can lead to an increase in ROM. It is important to do stretching and flexibility every day and will only take seconds to perform. Many exercises incorporate stretching and flexibility in their routine like warm-ups, Yoga, Pilates, calisthenics, plyometrics, and cool-downs are a combination of flexibility and stretching used as part of a daily work-out. Stretching and flexibility is best done not before resistant exercises but after when your muscles and joints are warmed-up. In cardiovascular exercise or aerobic exercise, stretching is best done before your work-out.

Body composition is the ration of lean muscle verses body fat. More on this later.

Exercise Ideas

Training can start before you get out of bed and that is by laying on your back in bed with your arms resting on the side of your body and stretching your legs by first pointing the toes to the foot of the bed and holding that stretch for four to five seconds: repeat these two to three times. Do the same thing to the heels of the foot by pointing the heels to the foot of the bed and hold this stretch position for four to five seconds. Stretch only to a position of comfort then relax and repeat the stretching routine. Once this is done remain on your back and without bending the hips, try and bring your shoulders up off the bed stretching the muscles of the back towards your hips: repeating these two or three times. Now for your shoulders and while still laying down on your back, raise your hands and arms up over your chest and try and reach for the ceiling, bring them down to your side and do it again: repeat these two to three times. This should take about 2 to 3 minutes to perform if done slowly and repeated. As you start to get out of bed, do this slowly until you are in a sitting position and once in a sitting position those of us that have problems getting in and out of bed or a chair this is a good time to exercise your hips, knees, ankles, and to control your balance. If you use a walker or a cane O.K. us it; I want you to stand up straight with good posture keeping your eyes open and looking straight-ahead then sit back down slowly on the bed, repeat these two to three times or more before moving away from the bed. This should take about 1 to 2 minutes so your total time spent doing these morning routines stretching exercises would be approximately 3 or 4 minutes and you never left the bedroom. By adding a slight twist to your sitting routine while still sitting on the bed is a good idea. While sitting with your back straight, slowly turn your chest to the right wall as much as comfort allows then slowly bring your back forward in front of you, again turn your chest to the left as much as comfort allows then return chest to the front. Repeat this as much as you feel capable of doing without discomfort. Do the same to the head with the chest remaining forward; turn your head to the right then bring it forward then turn your head to the left as much as comfort allows then bring the head forward, repeat these 2 to 3 times. Next stretch is with your chin and bring it forward touching the chest then back up and look straight head then bring your head backwards to look at the ceiling as comfort allows. Repeat these 2 to 3 times as long as no discomfort is present. There are other exercises that can be done but this will get you started.

Walking as an Aerobic Exercise

Exercise can be accomplished in many ways and it does not have to be strenuous although spending an hour in a gym is a good way to motivate the esprit de corps, meet new people, increase your circle of friends, and just to get out and walk. Most physical fitness books seem to just target the young and do not really venture into the more senior members of our society. If we have not been very active or have been active and just slowed down our activity as time crept into our lives, this must be taken into consideration. As such, starting an exercise program should be taken at a slow pace and in moderation. As a senior member, a complete physical examination is in order before embarking on this journey. Your doctor should be aware of your desire to become more physically active, in fact, your doctor should know exactly what type of physical activity you plan on venturing into **anaerobic, aerobic, or both** activities because the doctor's physical examination would be geared towards that goal. Follow your doctors advise as to the pros and cons of what you can do or cannot do.

Most doctors will recommend a good brisk walk. Walking is a good aerobic exercise and is one of the best exercises for the reduction of stressors from the everyday problems that accumulate daily. It will help you to mentally decompress and relax the nerves and tighten muscles after a long hard day not to mention a great way to lose weight. What is great about walking is that you need no equipment and it can be accomplished at any time. It is a low-level exercise routine that puts very little pressure on the hips, knees, ankles, and spine with very little bouncing movement involved minimizing muscle stress to all body parts. For the young, 50 and below years of age, walking is just a thing to get from point A to point B or more like a need than an exercise. The health benefits of walking do not always register with some because they have no real understanding of what exercise really is and when to used its fullest potential. "If you're not sweating, you're not exercising" is the common belief with the young and most fitness instructors. This is not true! Walking is an exercise and as long as you are doing the walking in earnest and as a fitness modality, you are accomplishing the goal and it's going to be of benefit. That means walking with the total mind, body, and spirit that this walk is for your health improvement and for the increase your endurance. Many will say that the calories burned when one walks a mile or jogs a mile is minimal to none but I disagree, I say that some calories being burned is better than no calories being burned and walking 10 or more minutes is better than lounging at home watching TV or doing nothing and performing no activities at all at home. In my building and on my floor, we have a long hallway which is about 28 yards long (84 feet) which goes from east to west and I have used the hallway for my walk numerous times as well as the stairs. You can even use the hallway if you have a walker or use a cane. If these items are needed it is strongly advised that you perform this walk with a partner present.

Aerobic Exercise Options

Depending on the speed of the walk, distance walked, and the duration (F.I.T.) of the walk will determine how many calories are actually burned. Speed of walking does not have to only be with an increase in gait or pace. One can increase the length of their stride or by widening their walking stance. Please do not only perform a walking exercise routine for the sole purpose of losing weight but if that is your motivation, go for it. Do it for the health benefit it presents; strengthening the heart, increasing respiratory volume, increase in muscle tone and strength with the added joint movement lubrication, as well as, the strengthening of the bones and an increase in endurance. As you continue this scheduled routine of walking, your heart and lungs will start to work less hampered and depending on how often you walk per week, this will make your cardiovascular system stronger and work a lot more efficiently. Burning more calories is a secondary contribution to walking. As you continue to walk or increase to a faster pace or jog per minute there will be an increase in respiratory and cardiac output as well as circulatory improvement which after a few weeks you will notice an increase, smoothness, and ease in your walking pace. Increasing speed of your pace does not always cause a great change in the number of calories burned but one will start to burn the calories in the body and cardiovascular system at a much faster rate than at a slower rate. At a moderate to brisk walking pace in 30 minutes a rule of thumb is one can burn around 100 to 200 or more calories per mile for a 180lb person. These calories being burned in the first 30 minutes will come from sugars stored in the body and if you continue to walk stored fat will start to be burned as fuel. Please keep in mind that even if you do not always walk for 30 minutes but walk for a shorter period time, you will still benefit from a good walk and yes, it is O.K. to walk every day if that is your decision.

Aerobic Dancing

Aerobic Dancing is another way of exercising and receiving a good cardiac workout. It is important, first, to understand what is meant by the word "aerobics" and or "aerobic metabolism." Aerobics means "requiring free oxygen" which is the use of oxygen for the demands needed by the body during the intensity of physical activities for an extended period of time. It refers to the use of fats and carbohydrates to continue its activities or aerobic metabolism. This word "Aerobic dancing" came about after World War II when physical activities like jogging started to become popular through the concept of a physical therapist Colonel Pauline Potts and Dr. Kenneth Cooper of the United States Air Force. They noticed the health benefits of jogging and running that came from this fitness activity. Dr. Cooper started to research this trend as a preventive medicine possibility. He was the first to cultivate and use the word "Aerobic Exercise" to identify this health benefits that was going on with the U.S. Air Force personnel. Dr. Cooper, in 1968, published his ideas in a book intitled **"Aerobics"** and in a newer version of his book in 1970 **"The New Aerobics"** he defines aerobic exercise as "the ability to use the maximum amount of oxygen during exhaustive work" (Wikipedia – Aerobic Exercise). Dr. Kenneth Cooper is now known as "The Father of Aerobics." I thought that you should understand the history of aerobics before I get into Aerobic Dancing.

Dance for Health

When referring to Aerobic Dancing or Aerobic Workout, it is important to know that it is also a fun way to perform a vigorous cardiovascular physical workout with the aid of music as a motivating initiator. You do not need to buy any CDs or DVDs to perform aerobic dancing, just turn on your radio to some music and start gyrating and dance to the rhythm. There is just one thing you need to know; Aerobic Dancing or workout requires that the whole body must be in constant motion for a period of time that's why it's called – **AEROBICS.** Aerobic is unlike anaerobic exercise because anaerobic exercise is a strength exercise program that does not improve to the fullest the efficiency of the endurance capabilities of the cardiovascular system and is not meant for this purpose, so in essences does not last long as an aerobic function. Anaerobic workout is more characterized as an exercise with the lack of oxygen that is available to the muscles and is a non-endurance type of sport endeavor but it does promote strength, speed, and power. To put it simply, aerobic and anaerobic exercise are different in the duration and the intensity of the muscular contractions as well as the energy that is generated by the muscles. Getting back to Aerobic Dancing; the practice and idea of Aerobic Dancing is not a new concept. It has been practiced, developed, and applied for thousands of years; it just was not called Aerobic Dancing. Kata's, shadow boxing, sword practice, punching the heavy bag, are all a form of this exercise concept and modality.

The origin of the name Aerobic Dancing can be traced back to a naval pilot's wife who started an exercise class in Puerto Rico in 1969. Her name was Jacki Sorenson and it was an exercise class with dancing that she called Aerobic Dancing because she used music with her exercise program. The music made the exercise fun unlike straight physical activity. Playing different song compilations inclusion made every exercise session different, enjoyable, and it changed the exercise dancing rhythm. Mrs. Sorenson started with calisthenics as the first type of music exercise that was done than with other musical movements added later, twists and gyrations became part of the fun that ensued. Aerobic Dancing started to spread as an exercise form to other military bases then to the public. In the 1970s Aerobic dancing become popular worldwide and in the 1980s it especially spread when Jane Fonda released her video version around 1982. Now a myriad of different music and forms of aerobic dancing has crept onto the scene of Aerobic Dancing and it is now even done in the swimming pools. Their forms of Aerobic Dancing are high impact, low impact, and non-impact with weights on ankles, waist or wrist, and many other creations of this. The question in everyone's mind is "Does Aerobic Dancing qualify as an **Aerobic exercise**" and "does it actually work to improving the cardiovascular system." Let just say this, according to studies on aerobic dancing exercises and the research that was done the answer is "Yes." Using the basic criteria, Aerobic Dancing does qualify as aerobic exercise as long as it follows the general principles of exertion; frequency, intensity, and time/duration. **Frequency** refers

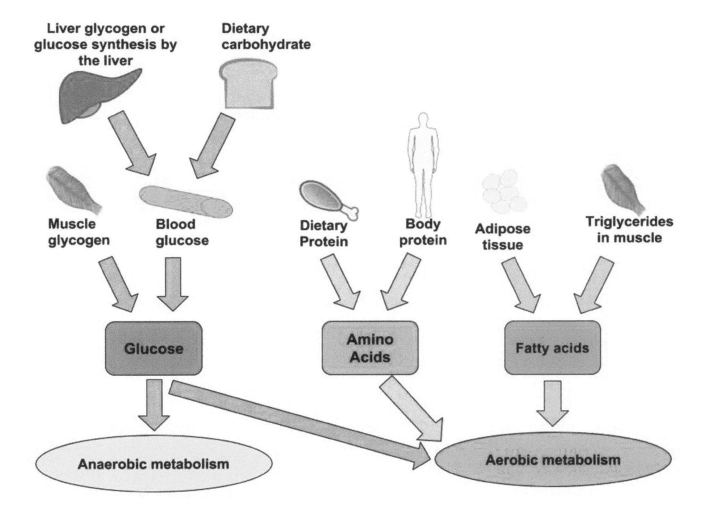

The difference between aerobic exercise and anaerobic exercise via the metabolic processes.

to the number of occurrences or times that you repeat the same function; in this case, the number of repetitive times done. It can also mean the number of movements done. **Intensity** refers to the quality of the force used and that means the strength, energy of feeling that is put into it and in this case the movement activities. **Time** refers more to how many or how often one puts into the workout or the duration spent, so Frequency = 4 times a week, Intensity = slow dancing to gradual increase in or the addition of weights, Time = the length of time spent on each dance routine that is 10, 20, 30, or 40 minutes per session. When using F.I.T., it will qualify as aerobic dancing or exercise because the activities can enhance cardiac stamina, muscle endurance, combined with skeletal fitness. Aerobic Dancing is very popular these days and numerous CDs and DVDs are sold on the market. I would like to suggest this before deciding on purchasing one. If you're new at Aerobic Dancing please start with music on the radio, to a slow rhythm first, and work up from there. Just like any physical activity, injuries can occur with Aerobic Dancing, in fact, when it first was introduced to the public there were many injuries that plagued aerobic dancing so pick a CD or DVD that has been reviewed by a physiologist or medical specialist (not all performers are qualified trainers in the field). A team of physiologist, in the early days, have helped to improve the fundamentals of this exercise dimension so that it can be adapted to all participants to use. As the population increased for the desire in aerobic dancing exercise there was a dynamic outspread of aerobic dancing concepts with many other movement exercises added that contribute to aerobic physical health, for instance, Zumba, Pilates, Tae Bo, and BodyPump and they all featured excellent physical training development programs.

Zumba fitness was started by a Colombian dancer Alberto "Beto" Pérez in the 1990s and basically consist of a core of 16 steps to the rhythm of: salsa, reggaeton, merengue, and cumbia with each basic rhythm having a core of four steps. They are approximately an hour long and are taught by a licensed Zumba fitness instructor. There are 10 types of exertion level classes for different ages and levels of training individuals. There is a lot more to this fitness program so study it first.

Pilates consists of low-level impact for the purpose of flexibility, strengthening of muscles, and endurance exercises. It emphasizes the alignment of the body and the balancing and strengthening of muscles throughout the body's core. It was first introduced in the 1920s by Joseph Pilates which he called Contrology.

Tae Bo is a fitness system that includes martial arts as part of a total physical workout routine. It incorporates kicks and punches in a rapid pace fitness design. It was first developed in 1976 by Billy Blanks concept of combining dance routines with elements of the martial arts (Taekwondo) and the merging of boxing techniques together to form Tae Bo. In the 1990s Tae Bo became popular when a series of videos were marketed to the public.

Aerobics Clarified

We have discussed what is meant by aerobics and it is now important to point out some salient points at this time. Not all formal aerobic classes follow the true concept of Aerobic Dancing and like the above exercise fitness programs, there are many with different names that use the name aerobic workout or Aerobic Dancing for their form of classes. A true Aerobic movement or dance class will be an exercise class that has their members in constant motion and this movement or motion will be of the total body type, legs, and arms. It is a whole-body movement that makes it an aerobic exercise to music. The intensity and frequency of this total movement must raise your heart rate and lung rate up, to increase vascular flow and the ability to hold that rate flow time for a specific duration for it to benefit the cardiovascular system. As we age our cardiovascular threshold changes its ability to tolerate variations in our physical capability. What took you 30 minutes to reach a good cardiovascular workout in 10 minutes years ago may take you 25 or 20 minutes to reach the same good cardiorespiratory workout. If you're not in constant motion, your heart would not be able to reach or increase its pulse and/or respiratory rate. Remember: Aerobics is the goal.

Cycling and other Exercises for Health and Fitness

We are all aware of the health benefits of cycling and doing this exercise on a regular basis can stimulate and improve the cardiovascular/cardiorespiratory system. Cycling can strengthen the heart, increase endurance, help reduce weight, increase muscle strength and stamina while it decreases stresses, anxiety, and depression just like walking and Aerobic Dancing can do. What is also interesting about cycling is that it is low-impact and causes less strain on the ankles, knees, and hips then most forms of aerobic activities. What I like most about cycling is that it can improve balance and coordination which prevents falls and possible fractures while still strengthening the leg muscles. What is good about cycling is that you do not have to ride a bicycle in the streets to develop these benefits. The one bad thing about cycling is that if you are not a member of a gym, the cost of a stationary bicycle can be quite expensive. To buy a stationary bicycle may range from 200 to 600 dollars or more and then you need to determine what type of stationary bike you want; a recumbent stationary bike or a regular seated cycle bike. You would be getting the same type of health benefits received from a street bike or a stationary bike or a stationary recumbent bike which is so much more comfortable to use but more expensive to buy. Other cardio exercises are the treadmill and the elliptical exercise machine as well as the rowing machine and all three will provide a good workout. The rowing machine is the hardest and the elliptical machine may require more balance and energy expenditure then the treadmill but the treadmill would provide a much more even distribution and rate of movement for a better walk or jog motion and is preferred as a potential choice for those that need the extra balance and coordination.

Strength Training and the Older Population

Strength training for the older adult population is just as important as it would be for any age group. It plays a major role in building and rebuilding muscle cells, strengthening muscle mass and increases tone, sustaining stamina, increasing the circulatory flow, increasing bone density, and just for the overall maintenance function of the body. No one is too old to start some sort of resistance exercise. Most of us start to loss body mass at or about the age of 30 or 40 and with this body mass is lost; bone density, strength, stamina, and endurance is also lost. Normal aging requires maintaining as much body mass as possible and this requires a regime of cardio and strength training to uphold a good sound inner core. To do this, we must hold onto as much of our youth as possible.

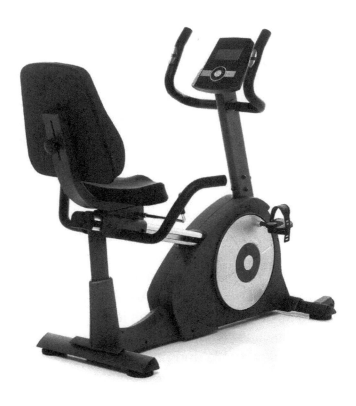

Recumbent Stationary Cycle

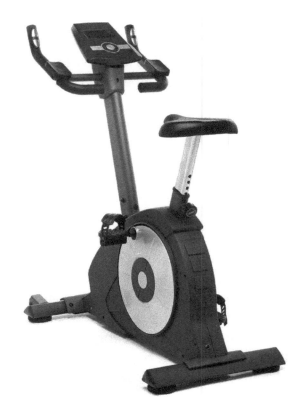

Stationary Cycle

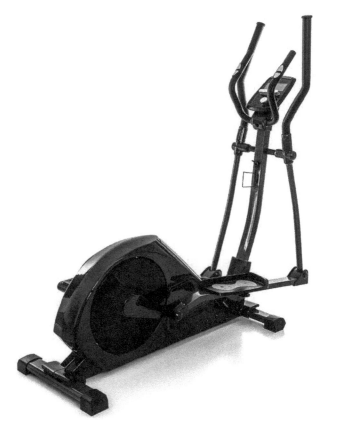

Elliptical Machine

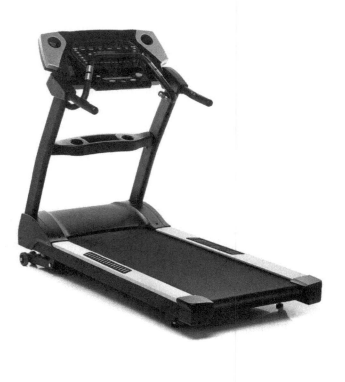

Treadmill machine

When we talk about strength training, we are talking about weight lifting which is an important exercise in maintaining the health of the bones and the prevention of osteoporosis which is one of the contributing factors in frailty. Strength training, as does cardio training, has been proven through research to be a safe and effective means to preserve a physically sound independent individual of all ages throughout the years.

There is a pamphlet written by **TUFTS: Nutrition and the CDC** called **"Growing Stronger: Strength Training for Older Adults,"** by Rebecca A. Seguin, B.S., CBCS & Jacqueline N. Epping, M.ED., written in 1998-2002 that can be obtained on your PC website free that goes into details regarding strength training for older adults. It is a must read for seniors and actually all ages in learning about strength training. There are those that believe as we age the loss of vital energy, mass, and strength does not have to apply if we use resistance training and cardio training on a routine basis. Their concept is "use it or lose it." This is partly true especially when it comes to the flexibility and mobility category. May I remind you that this loss is going to happen no matter how fit, trim, and athletic you are. We can, however slow it down. The aging process and time will march on.

As I have mentioned previously, we do not have to stand by and accept this aging process in its totality, you can greatly slow down this process and all it requires is that out of a 24-hour day leave open an hour for physical training. This essay was not meant to go into the total didactic learning course in the use of all the resistance training curriculum but there are certain terms and principles that one should be aware of. There are two basic types of resistance training perceptions and that is **"push and pull"** and this will cause **flexions and extensions** of the joints specifically to the push or pull muscles, tendons, and joints. Flexion will cause the muscles to contract **(prime movers)** and this will shorten the angle of the joint bringing the bones or limbs together. This is called **(concentric contraction or agonist).** Extension **(eccentric contraction or antagonistic)** does the opposite of contraction or prime movers so as the muscle contract the extenders lengthen getting ready to return the limb to its starting position.

Push or pull – Push is when you lift weights away from the body. Pull is when you bring the weights towards the body.

Flexion and extension – Flexion or bending movement around the joints that decreases the angle between the bones of the limbs at the joint. Extension is the unbending movement around joints in a limb that increasing the angle between the bones of the limb at the joint.

Muscle contractions (Prime mover) – Prime movers is the shortening or thickening of the muscle fiber. There are many forms of muscle contractions:

- ✓ **Agonist** or the muscle action that shortens the muscle fiber.
- ✓ **Antagonist** or the muscle action that works to bring or return the limb to its original position. It is the opposite to contraction/agonist.

Antagonistic Muscle Groups

Muscles work in groups and in pairs to form a complete action potential matrix – one muscle or prime muscle contracts the opposite of the other muscle extends then it is reversed, the extender becomes the prime and the prime becomes the extender. This is what is called antagonistic muscle groups; working together but in opposite contention to the other. Here is an example of antagonistic muscle groups:

1. **Pectoral muscles – Latissimus dorsi**
2. **Anterior muscles – Posterior muscles**
3. **Left External Oblique's – Right External Oblique's**
4. **Quadriceps muscles – Hamstring muscles**
5. **Biceps muscles – Triceps muscles**
6. **Forearm flexors – Forearm extensors**

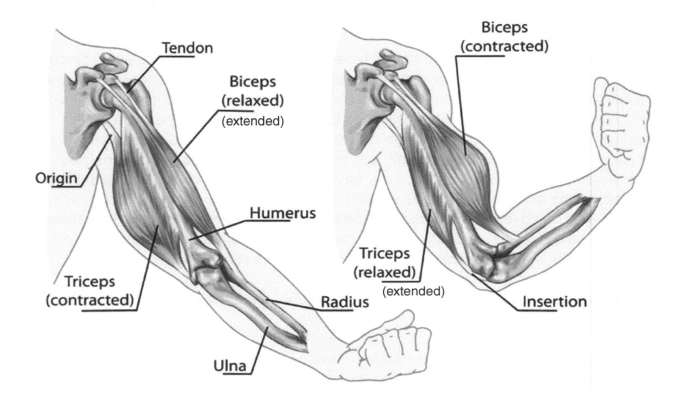

What the above means is when you contract the pectoral muscles you will lengthen the latissimus dorsi muscle and the latissimus dorsi muscle will bring the limb back to its original position, etc. Again, I cannot give a full didactic course in resistance or cardiovascular training but once you appreciate the value of being in a physically fit state of mind and body, it becomes part of your life and just seems to make living much more relaxing, less stressful, and a lot more enjoyable. Repeating what was already written: a good cardiovascular resistance workout on a routine and scheduled regiment will help to:

✓ Improve efficiency in daily activities
✓ Improve the cardiovascular system
✓ Improve the ability to control stress
✓ Improve your confidence
✓ Improve energy level for daily activities
✓ Improve your feeling of being in control of yourself

Have a physical examination by a physician before embarking on and physical exercise program. There are a number of changes that may have to be made if the desired results cardiovascular and/or resistance exercises are to be achieved for overall level of fitness. Even us old folks still have habits that must be weighed and measured with changes that may have to be made for the good of our self and our love one's. Some resistance exercises can actually be done at home using a quart, half gallon, and gallon containers of milk container with some water as weights, the floor or bed for sit-ups and the floor or wall for push-ups and you canuse the chair for squats. I am sure you can find other ways of performing resistance exercising at home; just use your imagination. Whatever exercise you start, you should maintain and continue it in a safe manner with good form and posture. There is no wrong way of exercising as long as it is a safe way.

A. **Do not over train**
B. **Exercise throughout the year**
C. **Relax during and after exercising and in your daily life**
D. **Eat a balanced meal**
E. **Maintain a reasonable weight or strive towards that goal**
F. **Do not smoke or abuse drugs**
G. **Alcohol should be avoided or consumed in moderation**
H. **Exercise will help you to relieve stress**
I. **Develop good sleeping habits**

Personally, going to a gym is a lot more enjoyable in encouraging you to in maintaining the will to exercise, meeting people, and just getting out of the house or the apartment and socializing. The atmosphere in the gym will put you in the mood to work the weights and learn about the equipment in the fitness center. Working with the equipment will give you a sense of accomplishment and when you leave the gym, you will feel the sense of fulfillment. Keep in mind that physical training is like a quid pro quo, whatever you put into your workout is what you will get out of your workout. Though I cannot give personal instructions on the use of the exercise equipment so using the old expression "A picture is worth a thousand words" it is with hope that these illustrations below will give you an idea as to the equipment that you may find and use or wish to use and the visual application of the apparatus you may encounter in most exercise centers. Bon appétit.

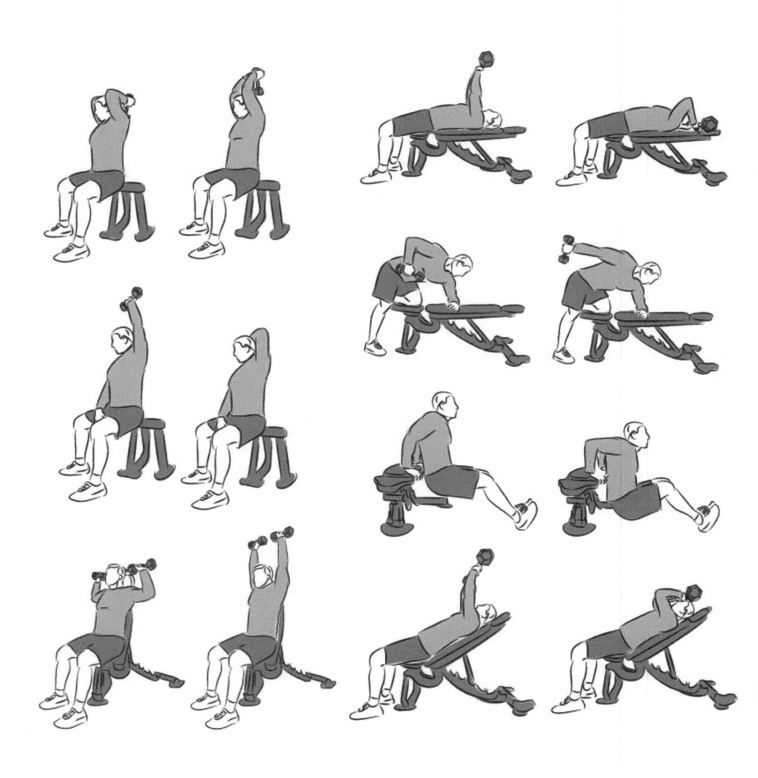

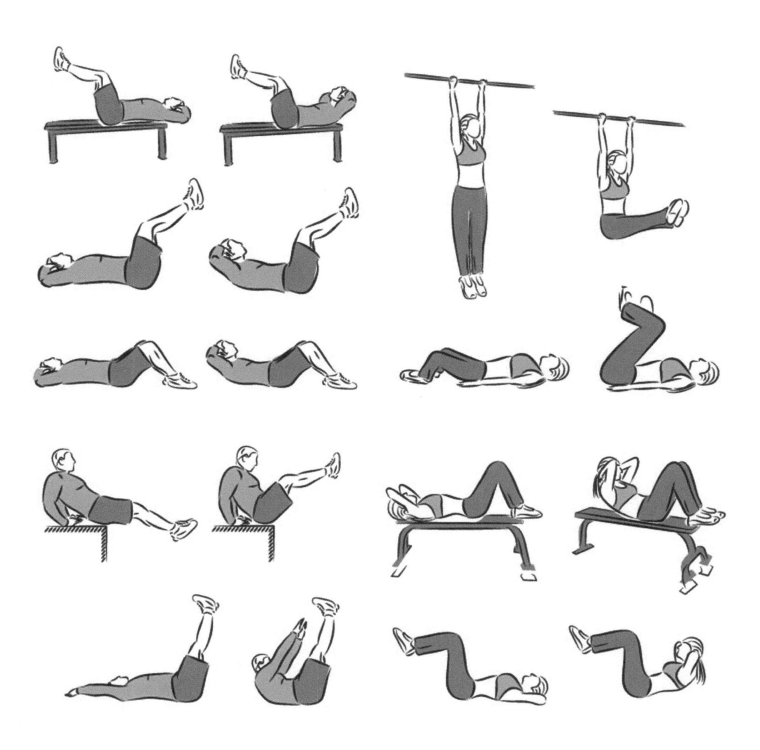

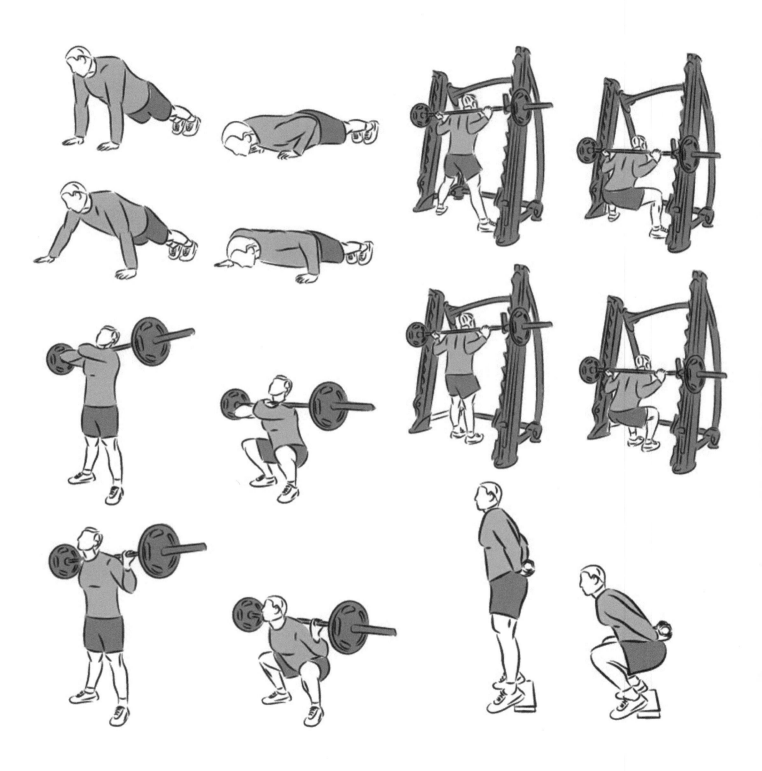

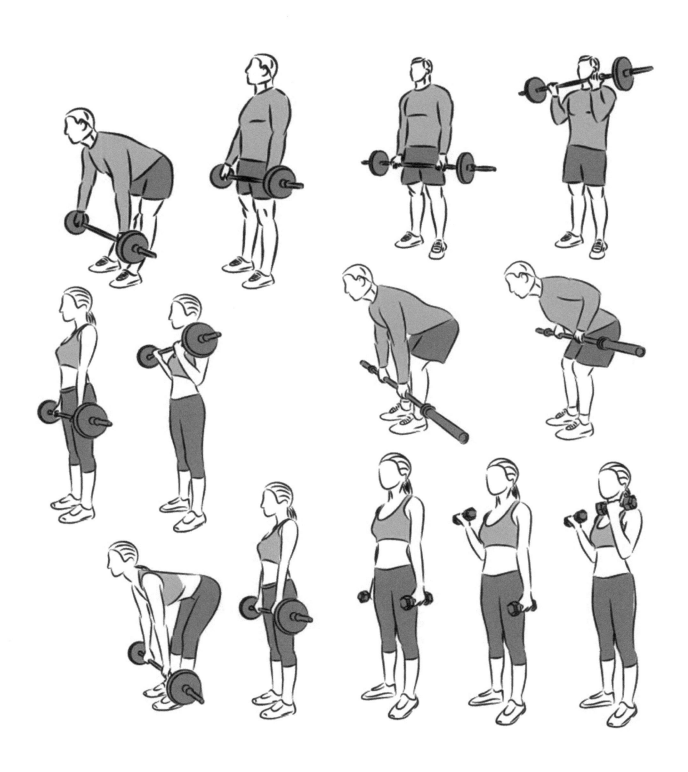

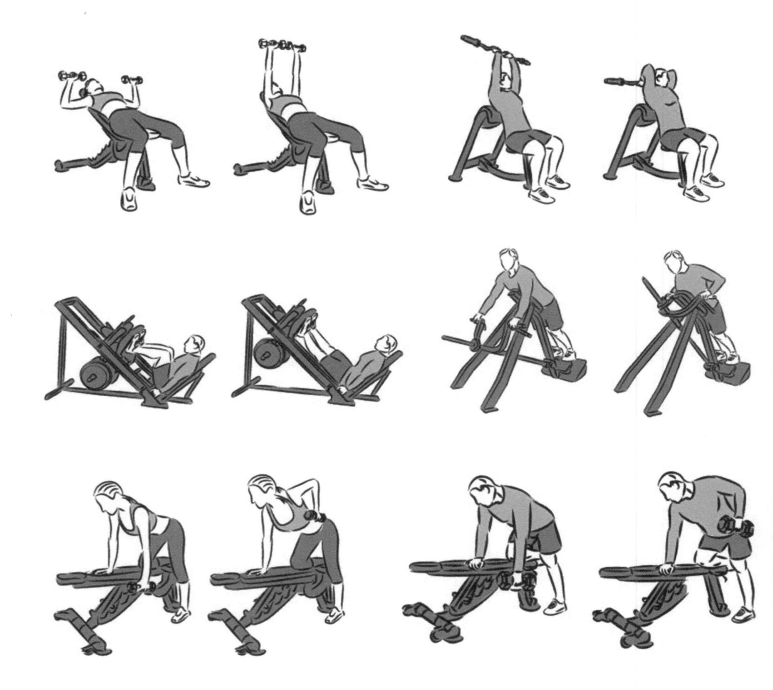

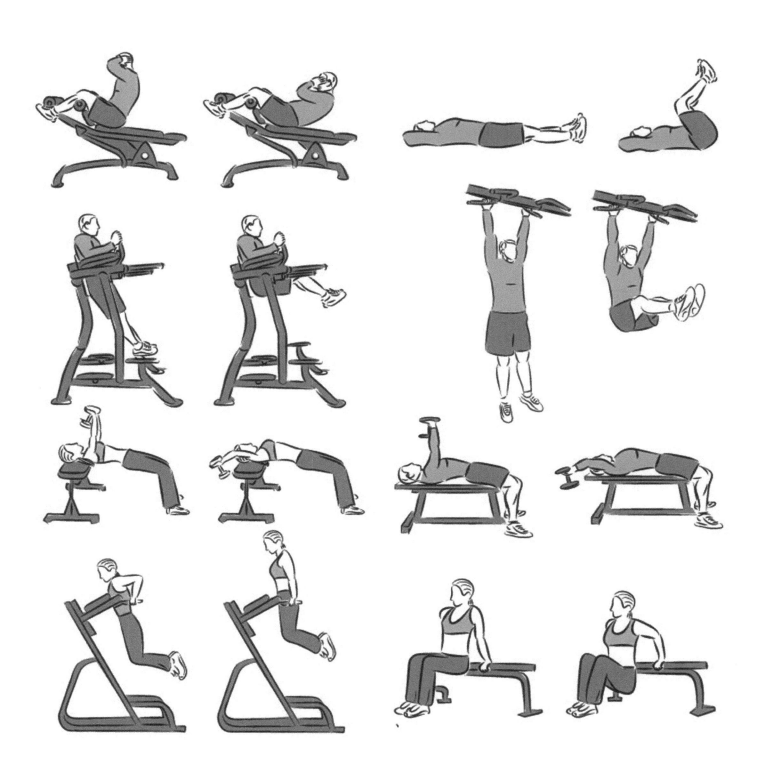

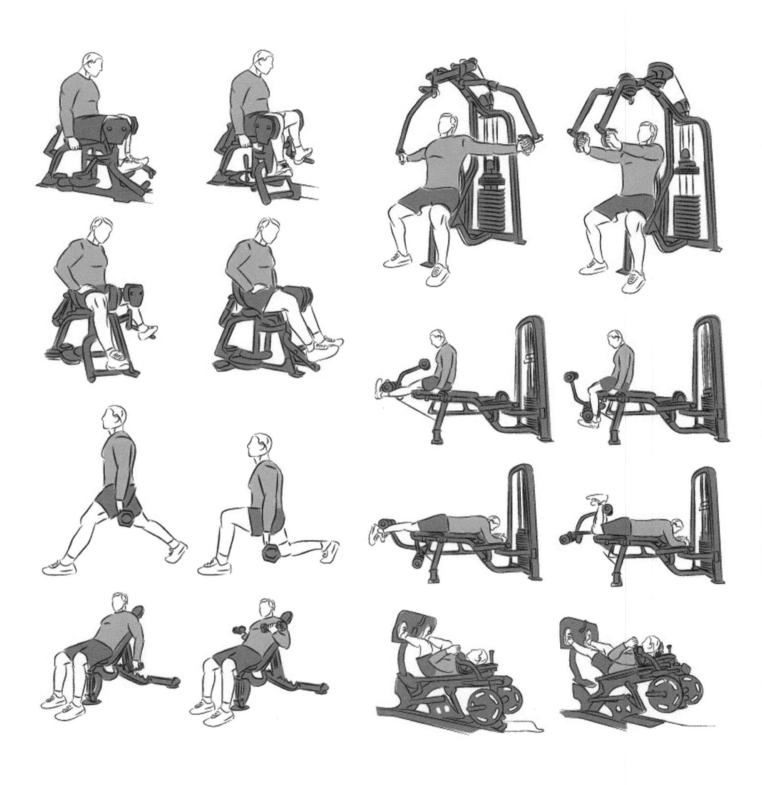

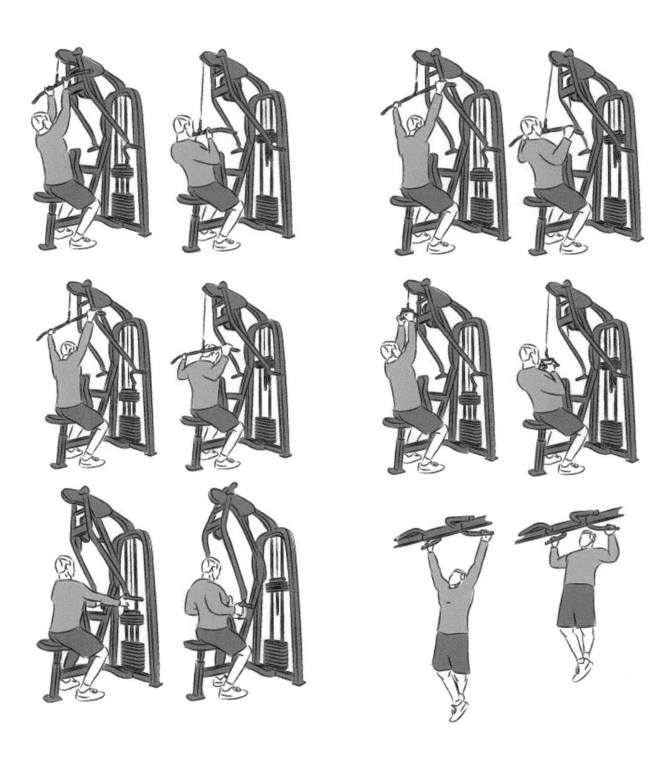

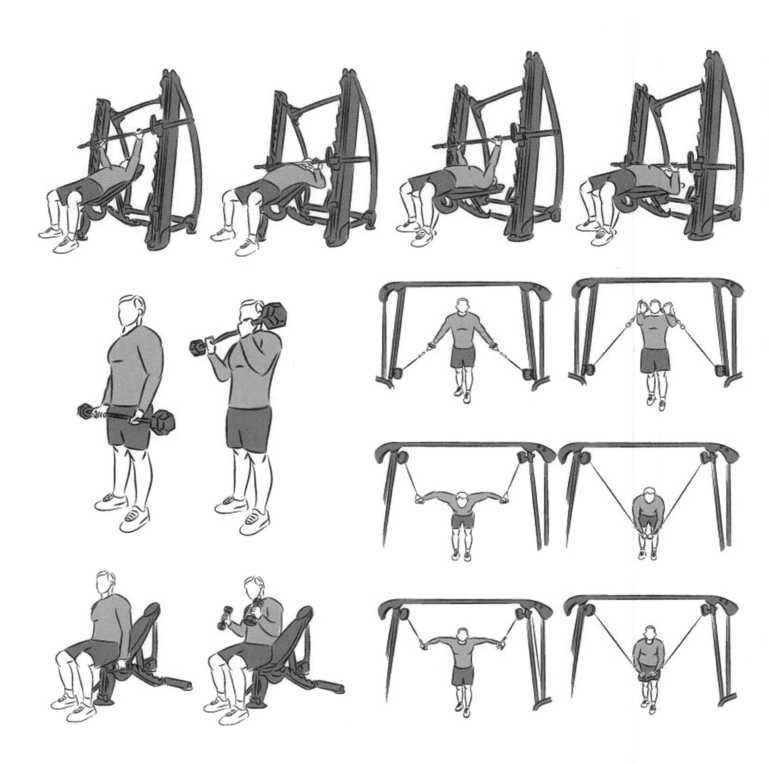

Record your exercise routines

Exercise Journal

Name: _____ Date: _____ Week: _____ Day: _____

CARDIOVASCULAR	LEVEL/PROGRAM	INTENSITY	DURATION/MINUTES
Check One	Circle One	Circle One	Check One
• Treadmill • Stair climber • Stationary Bike • Stationary Rower • Aerobics Step Class • Elliptical Trainer • Other_____	1 2 3 4 5 6 7 8 9 10 11 12 13 14 15 Other_____	Beats in 10 Seconds 15 16 17 18 19 20 21 22 23 24 25 26 27 28 29	••••• 0 - 15 ••••• 16 - 30 ••••• 31 - 45 ••••• 46 - 60 ••••• 61 - 75 ••••• 76 - 90

Weight Training										
REST BETWEEN SETS Seconds_____	Set #1		Set #2		Set #3		Set #4		Set #5	
EXERCISES	REPS	WT	REPS	WT	REPS	WT	REPS	WT	REPS	WT

Chapter 10

Weight Loss and the Older Population

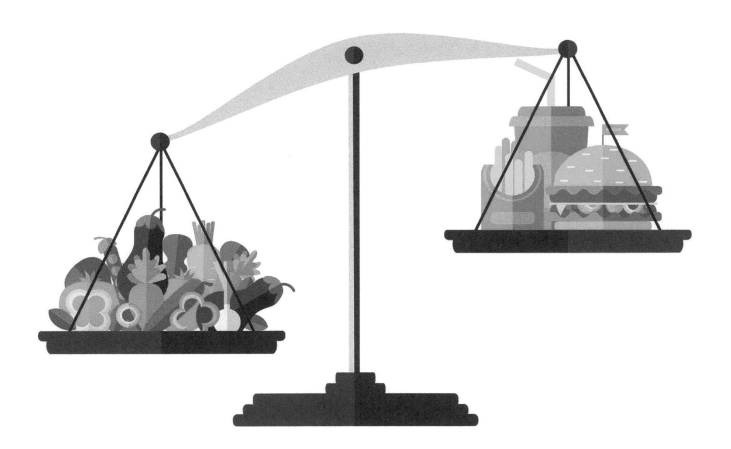

Contents in Chapter 10

Weight Loss and the Older Population

Losing weight has come under some scrutiny in this text as it relates to the older adults. It has been used as a scale to determine frailty, dementia, and just being unhealthy and not for the health of the person that is just trying to loss a few pounds. Yes, this can be a means of determining the health status of an individual that is losing weight without the intention of doing so and this can be interpreted with other causal risk factors as a prognostication of a health concerning event. This should not interfere with an older person's desire to just truly trying to loss those tell-tale signs of being overweight. As we become older, losing weight becomes much harder and more problematic biologically because the hormonal chemistry and the brain have excepted and are satiated and have settled on what is the present body weight. It does not rationalize as to what it can be. There are so many articles and remedies as to how one can loss weight that it all becomes a guesstimation as to which one of the articles to choose because they all sound so positive and one idea looks better then the other idea so the query is; which one can you afford to do. Not one of them tell you what you should really know about being overweight or what is important. That query is, "what the heck is fat and how important is it to my health." We all know the basic facts of what fat or **adipose** tissue which is that it functions as a source of stored energy for the body but that is it. It is now the time to fill in the gaps that are missing in the fat cell saga.

What are Lipids?

The average human has 30 billion fat cells weighing about 30lbs and we know that it is closely linked to the body mass index (BMI). This fatty tissue experiences happens rapidly during the toddler stage of life around the age of 2 and continues until adulthood where it slowly stops and stabilizes at age 16.5. In some individuals, the fat cells also called **adipocytes** will continue to rise until the age of 20 at which time it stabilizes and remains relatively constant. The fat cells are all created at youth will remain constant for a life time regardless of weight loss or gain. It is believed that the adult human cannot create new fat cells and the way fat cells increase in mass is by adding more lipids into the fat cell itself which in turn increases the weight of the cell. In Sweden, the research at Karolinska Institute and at Lawrence Livermore National Laboratory (LLNL) have demonstrated that in some cases one can create new fat cells regardless of their body weight, sex, or age. This still has to be researched to further its validity. At this time fat cells in the body are set during adolescence and remain the same in amount in the body throughout adulthood and once lifetime. Within the tissue itself there are numerous fat cell seeds that remain dormant but can be triggered to grow by hormones, diet, and inactivity of the individual. This is just a belief and is not set-in fact. Scientists have looked at fat cells in individuals that have had severe weight loss or gains of weight and it was determined that weight loss or gain was the result of a boost or loss in fat cell size and not in the number of fat cells itself. This basically means that weight loss was due to the fat cells shrinking but not vanishing and weight gain is due to fat cells fulling up with lipid fluids. This did not matter if the weight loss was after stomach-stapling surgery; the amount and number of fat cells remained the same after 2 years although the fat cells themselves have fewer fat lipids within the cells. This basically means that if you are overweight and lose this weight, the capacity to regain the weight back is within your mental capacity because biologically you still have the same number of fat cells. This is why it is so hard to lose weight. It is sometimes disturbing to see some friends that can eat just about anything and not gain any weight. This may be due to the fact that they have a low-fat cell count or number or that they have a very active metabolic system. Those that gain weight easily may be because they have a greater fat cell number than the so-called naturally slimmer person. Fat cells do die, as do all living cells, new fat cells are created to keep the amount of fats cells in the body at a constant and stabilized number. What should be understood is that all fat cells have the same weight and volume and it does not matter where the fat cells are distributed and/or located in the body. The concentration of fat cells depends on one's race and gender. Some men carry fat cells in their chest, abdomen, thighs, and buttocks areas of the body and females carry more fat cells in their breast, hips upper legs, waist, upper arms, and the buttocks region. Females tend to have more fat cells than men. These female fat cells are located in layers at strategic positions on the body and this difference in the location is due to the sex hormones estrogen and testosterone.

Genetics and Fat Cells

Genetics factors plays a role in the number of fat cells one has in a continuous mode but this is just 30 percent of the DNA coding influence and this can be superseded by the 70 percent that is controlled by the human factor. It has been said that once you become obese at a young age, fat cell numbers can increase regardless of the genetic possibilities. In other words, obesity at a young age can change the genetic matrix and the body fat cells count settled can become a much higher number than these fat cells would have been before the young body stabilized and this new induce amount now becomes a constant during your teenage and adult years. This means that the adult will have a greater number of fat cells to deal with in his or her older age group and so the battle for weight control is a possibility in later life. The genes will regenerate loss fat cells or it may increase the size of the fat cell itself. This may be the genes way of protecting the fat cells as it does for all the cells in the body to ensure continuity. Fat cells or adipose tissue do this by secreting a hormone called **leptin** and **enterocytes** that helps regulate energy balance inhibiting hunger which reduces fat cell storage in the adipocyte. This leptin triggers receptor cells in the **hypothalamus** which is the central location of the hunger center of the brain/body. Leptin hormone interacts with other hormones such as insulin, glucagon, growth hormones, cytokines, and other metabolites. Although leptin effects many hormones and organs systems it is important to note that studies in mice have shown that the administration of leptin can ameliorate certain brain pathologies and improve cognitive performance. Leptin has reduced beta-amyloid and hyperphosphorylated Tau which are the two trademarks of Alzheimer's disease. There is another hormone that you should be aware of called **ghrelin.** The name Ghrelin was derived from **g**rowth **h**ormone **rel**easing peptides discovered in 1999. Leptin helps to reduce your appetite but ghrelin increases your appetite. Ghrelin is produced in the **enteroendocrine** of the gastrointestinal tract but it is especially found in the stomach and duodenum, as well as, the lungs, pancreatic islets, and other organs of the body. It is known as the hunger hormone. This hormone is important because it prepares your stomach by increasing gastric secretions and motility or movement of the cilia muscles in the gastrointestinal tract. The ghrelin activates the **pituitary gland** as well as the **hypothalamic neuropeptide** region of the hypothalamus that initiating the appetite response. This hormone also participates in the cognition, memory, sleep and awareness patterns, taste, glucose, and other behavioral metabolic functions. A major function of ghrelin is that it regulates the complex process of energy homeostasis which means that it controls aspects of the energy input and output needed by the body, fat and glycogen storage, and regulates the amount of heat loss. The most important thing to get from all of this is that your body's homeostasis is continually being monitored as a result of its needs through these metabolic signals.

Maintaining Metabolic Fat Constance

The question that we should be asking is "how do we keep the fat cell numbers in a constant state of balance yet reduce the amount of lipids in the fat cell body." If you do not change the volume or size of the fat cells, you do not change weight of the individual. We have already answered this question a number of times, dieting, exercising, reducing stress, getting adequate sleep, and no smoking or alcohol. Antioxidants can play a role in reducing the number of unwanted fat cells in the circulatory system. This has been said ad-infinitum and yet a little more than half of the population in the United States are overweight. According to the CDCs statistics, 65.2 percent of the U.S. population is considered to be overweight or obese. This was determined by the BMI calculation that takes into consideration a person's height and weight and this has been a good way of determining a person's body fat percentage. It is important to understand that it does not matter what body type one has because we are subjected, eventually, to gaining weight either early or later in life. This weight gain can be from fluids or fats or living a more sententary lifestyle. Some of these trends are related to genetics, at least 30% of it is anyway. The other 70% is up to you. This does not mean that poor eating habits and low daily energy expenditures are not contributing factors because they definitely are a major part of the weight fluctuation. There are classifications of overweight or obesity that can be determined by using the BMI calculation charts derived from the American Health Association. One can use this as a quick glance reference to weight gain or loss, take or give 25lbs. There are many good BMI charts with much more detail on the internet that one can use like the one on the next page.

Classification of Obesity at a Quick Glance

Category	% percentage over ideal weight	Body mass index (kg/m²)	Prevalence % of total obese population in (U.S.)
Underweight		<18.5	
Normal		18.5-24-5	
Overweight	20-40	25-26.9	
Obese		27-29.9	
Moderately obese	41-100	30-34.9	90.5
Severely obese		35-39.9	9.0
Morbidly obese	> -100	>40	0.5

BODY MASS INDEX (BMI) CHART

Weight

| ft/in | cm | lbs 90 | 100 | 110 | 120 | 130 | 140 | 150 | 160 | 170 | 180 | 190 | 200 | 210 | 220 | 230 | 240 | 250 | 260 | 270 | 280 | 290 |
		kgs 41	45	50	54	59	64	68	72	77	82	86	91	95	100	104	109	113	118	122	127	132
4 ft 8 in	142.2	20	22	25	27	29	31	34	36	38	40	43	45	47	49	52	54	56	58	61	63	65
4 ft 9 in	144.7	19	22	24	26	28	30	32	35	37	39	41	43	45	48	50	52	54	56	58	61	63
4 ft 10 in	147.3	19	21	23	25	27	29	31	33	36	38	40	42	44	46	48	50	52	54	56	59	61
4 ft 11 in	149.8	18	20	22	24	26	28	30	32	34	36	38	40	42	44	46	48	51	53	55	57	59
5 ft 0 in	152.4	18	20	21	23	25	27	29	31	33	35	37	39	41	43	45	47	49	51	53	55	57
5 ft 1 in	154.9	17	19	21	23	25	26	28	30	32	34	36	38	40	42	44	46	47	49	51	53	55
5 ft 2 in	157.4	16	18	20	22	24	26	27	29	31	33	35	37	38	40	42	44	46	48	49	51	53
5 ft 3 in	160.0	16	18	19	21	23	25	27	28	30	32	34	35	37	39	41	43	44	46	48	50	51
5 ft 4 in	162.5	15	17	19	21	22	24	26	27	29	31	33	34	36	38	39	41	43	45	46	48	50
5 ft 5 in	165.1	15	17	18	20	22	23	25	27	28	30	32	33	35	37	38	40	42	43	45	47	48
5 ft 6 in	167.6	15	16	18	19	21	23	24	26	27	29	31	32	34	36	37	39	40	42	44	45	47
5 ft 7 in	170.1	14	16	17	19	20	22	24	25	27	28	30	31	33	34	36	38	39	41	42	44	45
5 ft 8 in	172.7	14	15	17	18	20	21	23	24	26	27	29	30	32	33	35	37	38	40	41	43	44
5 ft 9 in	175.2	13	15	16	18	19	21	22	24	25	27	28	30	31	33	34	35	37	38	40	41	43
5 ft 10 in	177.8	13	14	16	17	19	20	22	23	24	26	27	29	30	32	33	34	36	37	39	40	42
5 ft 11 in	180.3	13	14	15	17	18	20	21	22	24	25	27	28	29	31	32	33	35	36	38	39	40
6 ft 0 in	182.8	12	14	15	16	18	19	20	22	23	24	26	27	28	30	31	33	34	35	37	38	39
6 ft 1 in	185.4	12	13	15	16	17	18	20	21	22	24	25	26	28	29	30	32	33	34	36	37	38
6 ft 2 in	187.9	12	13	14	16	17	18	19	21	22	23	24	26	27	28	30	31	32	33	35	36	37
6 ft 3 in	190.5	11	13	14	15	16	18	19	20	21	23	24	25	26	28	29	30	31	33	34	35	36
6 ft 4 in	193.0	11	12	13	15	16	17	18	19	21	22	23	24	26	27	29	30	32	33	34	35	
6 ft 5 in	195.5	11	12	13	14	15	17	18	19	20	21	23	24	25	26	27	28	30	31	32	33	34
6 ft 6 in	198.1	10	12	13	14	15	16	17	18	20	21	22	23	24	25	27	28	29	30	31	32	34
6 ft 7 in	200.6	10	11	12	14	15	16	17	18	19	20	21	23	24	25	26	27	28	29	30	32	33
6 ft 8 in	203.2	10	11	12	13	14	15	16	18	19	20	21	22	23	24	25	26	27	29	30	31	32
6 ft 9 in	205.7	10	11	12	13	14	15	16	17	18	19	20	21	24	25	26	27	28	29	30	31	
6 ft 10 in	208.2	9	10	12	13	14	15	16	17	18	19	20	21	22	23	24	25	26	27	28	29	30
6 ft 11 in	210.8	9	10	11	12	13	14	15	16	17	18	19	20	21	22	23	25	26	27	28	29	30

Height

Legend: Underweight | Healthy | Overweight | Obese | Extremely Obese

To calculate your BMI, multiply your weight in pounds by 703, and then divide the results by your height in inches squared. For example, if your height is 5feet 9inches or 69inches tall and your weight is around 180lbs:

$$180 \times 703 = 126,560$$
$$(69^2)\ 69 \times 69 = 4,761$$
$$126,540 \div 4,761 = 26.578$$

BODY MASS INDEX

UNDERWEIGHT	NORMAL	OVERWEIGHT	SEVERE OBESITY	MORBID OBESITY	SUPER OBESITY
< 18.5	18.5 - 24.5	25 - 30	35 - 39.5	40 - 44.5	45 - 50

In order to better understand fat cells or adipose tissue, one must know that there are two types of fat cells, white adipose tissue (WAT) and brown adipose tissue (BAT).

- **White fat cells or white adipose tissue (also known as body fat) (WAT),** are important for energy metabolism, maintaining body heat, and is used as a cushion. It contains a single large fat droplet which forces the nucleus to be squeezed to the periphery of the cell wall membrane. There are receptors for various hormones such as insulin, sex hormones, norepinephrine, and glucocorticoids. It also acts as a thermal insulator to maintain body temperature. This is the primary area where **leptin** is produced and **asprosin** (a protein hormone).

- **Brown fat cells or brown adipose tissue (BAT),** contain many mitochondria's and many large oily droplets that are smaller than the white fat cells oily droplets. It is not as common as the white fat cells but is present more in physically active individuals then in the less active and sedentary person. As humans become older, these brown fat cells decrease in number. The BATs primary function is **thermoregulation** and heat production by the muscles during shivering and **thermogenesis** when muscles are not shivering. The brown fat cells have more capillaries and are supplied with more oxygen and nutrients then the white fat cells. The brown fat cells have much more mitochondria and it is these mitochondria's that give the fat cells its brown color.

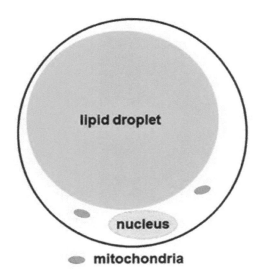

White Fat
Energy Storage

lipid droplet

nucleus

mitochondria

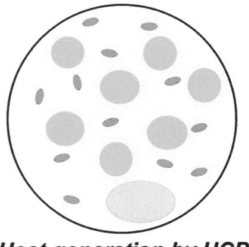

Brown Fat
Energy Burning*

Heat generation by UCP1

Please be aware that the BMI calculation percentage does not necessarily mean that the person with a high index faces a higher unhealthy risk factor and those that have a low index are heathier. It becomes of some concern when fat cells are stored around internal organs especially the upper portion of the body. Fats are needed in the body as a lubricant and it is an important constituent for the membranes of cells, to make hormones as well as a storage area for fat soluble vitamins. The body also uses adipocytes to transmit messages throughout the body. There are concerns and health hazards of being obese and these health hazard worries are well known.

Fat and the Diet

Losing weight should be simple; less calories and more exercise equals a reduction in weight. Yet, it just isn't that easy. Fats enter the body when you eat foods that contain these fats and triglycerides and once in the body they are then broken down into fatty acids. This breakdown starts from the munched bolus in the mouth mixing with the saliva. The saliva contains enzymes such as amylase, salivary lipase, and other enzymes that break down this bolus to a molecular level and this continues in the stomach and the intestines. When fat cells enter the body, it becomes adipocytes.

1. This process starts with bile salts from the gallbladder and this process is called **emulsification.** This bile continues to mix digesting the munch until it has broken it down to droplets called **micelles** which increases the fats surface area.

2. Enzymes secretions from the pancreas called lipases mixes with the micelles and breaks the fat further to glycerol and fatty acids that are then absorbed through the intestines.
3. Once absorbed they are reunited as a fat molecule (ATP) with a protein coating called **chylomicrons** which helps the fat dissolve better.
4. This ATP is released into the lymphatic system where they are stored because they are too large to go into the capillary bloodstream.
5. The veins and the lymphatic system now can allow the chylomicrons ATP to enter the blood stream where the chylomicrons are eventually eliminated and the enzyme lipoprotein lipases breaks down the fat into fatty acids.

It will never happen that all fat cells one gains can be eliminated because our genes are programmed to have a specific number of fat cells. Scientist are still not sure why some people have more fat cells than others or why women exhibit more adipose tissue than men although the primary theory or explanation is the hormones. What we do know is that fat cells in the human body is an excellent and convenient way to carry a large storage supply of potential energy and keep in mind that it is one of the basic building blocks of energy and food.

What is White Adipose Tissue (WAT)?

Those of us that have had to go on a weight reducing program for health reasons or a diet restriction watch list be it for personal appearance motives or modesty concerns such as those unsightly cellulite worries on the thighs, hips, buttocks, stomach, and arms or to get rid of that pudginess around the belly region, one can understand the frustration of hard work with little results. Fat is necessary for survival; the trick is balancing this fat in our everyday lives with diet, exercise, and just plain common sense. I wish I knew this a lot earlier in my life. The question is what and where is this adipose tissue? That's easy, it's in the organ called skin and around ever other body organ. Adipose tissue is under the subcutaneous area of the skin and throughout the body. One fatty cell is called adipocyte and the body contains millions of them.

ADIPOCYTE

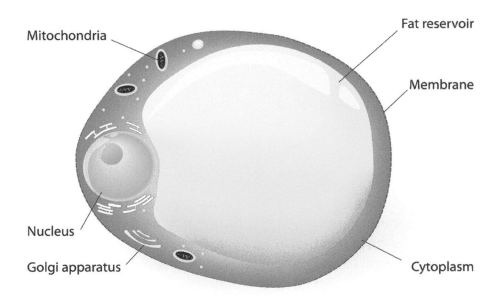

Not only is it used as a potential storage source as energy for the body, it is used as padding or cushioning and generates hormones that the body needs called **adiponectin's** which regulate insulin production. Adipose tissue is considered a major endocrine organ. It is ironic but the fatter one is the less adiponectin's the fatty cells produce. This can be problematic for the pancreas and insulin regulation which can trigger heart disease and diabetes. Osama Hamby, MD, PhD of Harvard Medical School has reported that visceral fat (fat around the abdomen) is toxic because it secretes an inflammatory protein called cytokines that have a direct effect on insulin production raising the risk of type 2 diabetes. He continues to say that under MRI or a CT scan, this can actually be seen. To measure this without the use of equipment, one just has to measure around the midsection of the waistline and if the reading is 35 inches or more there is a possibility that you have this visceral fat.

STRUCTURE OF THE SKIN

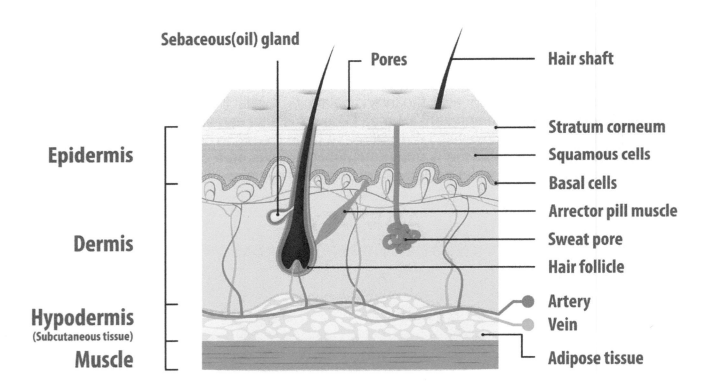

Sebaceous(oil) gland
Pores
Hair shaft
Stratum corneum
Squamous cells
Basal cells
Arrector pill muscle
Sweat pore
Hair follicle
Artery
Vein
Adipose tissue

Epidermis
Dermis
Hypodermis
(Subcutaneous tissue)
Muscle

What is Brown Adipose Tissue (BAT)?

Brown adipose tissue was once considered present only in infants and young children and that this BAT gradually disappears. In resent research (2009), studies have shown that this was not the case. Some adults still have this brown fat cells. Brown fat cells can be located around the neck, supraclavicular area (collarbone), shoulder blades, along the spinal cord, and chest. There is a beige fat cells similar to the brown fat cells that does not have as many mitochondria. Brown fat cells become active when the body is exposed to cold temperatures because it generates heat burning up energy to warm the body. BAT is the **thermoregulatory** of the body. White cells can be triggered to act like brown cells by exposing a person in the cold with temperatures below 60 degrees for 15 to 20 minutes; the white fat cells will produce a hormone called **irisin.** One can get this same effect from an hour of moderate exercise in a warm gym. Exercise is a great equalizer when it come to the body fat balance determination of constants and internal biological dynamic development.

There is another way of determining if you are carrying too much fat. Of courses, you can have a BMI done or have a Physical Trainer do a "The Skin Pinch Test" which is a skin caliper measurement test on you. This is done by measuring the fat folds via pinching specific areas of the body and measuring the folds. There are two good pinch tests, the 7-body fat fold pinch test and the 3-body fat fold pinch test. In the 3-body fat pinch test the upper arm, thigh, and stomach are measured and in the 7-body fat pinch test the arm, thigh, stomach, triceps, calf, abdomen, and iliac crest are pinched and measured. Although there are more than 7 illustrations shown choose the 7 mention.

Standard Skinfold Sites

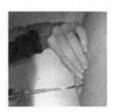
Triceps

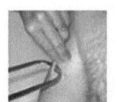
Biceps

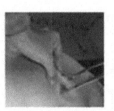
Subscapular

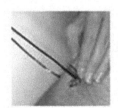
Thigh

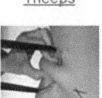
Iliac Crest

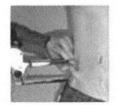
Supraspinale

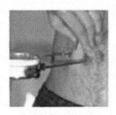
Abdominal

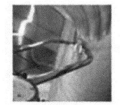
Calf

Other Traditional Sites

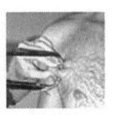
Chest

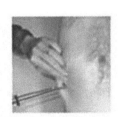
Axilla

You can buy skin calibrators at most pharmacy stores. Another way of determining body fat is through an at home bioelectrical impedance scale. There are two types, one that you stand on like a regular weight scale and one that you grab with two hands and hold for a few seconds. It works by sending an electrical current through your body and measures the speed in which it leaves your body. It is pretty accurate. Again, your friendly neighborhood pharmacy should have these items. There are other more complicated methods but these are the simples.

Cellulite in a Nutshell

Cellulites is a common but harmless condition of the skin associated with dimples and lumpiness, highs and lows of the thighs, hips, buttocks, and the abdomen but It can also appear on your breast and upper arms. It is not just associated with women but men as well. No one really knows why this happens but we do know the physiology that causes the condition. It is the fat in the subcutaneous connective tissue that herniates peripherally that causes the dimpling of the skin. This happens to 85 to 98% of women in postpubescent age group. It is thought to be a heredity and/or hormonal condition which includes metabolism, diet, obesity, genetic, and a host of other physiological factors that may predispose one to this condition.

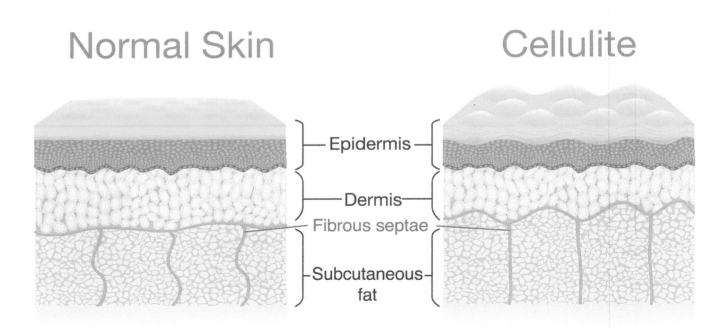

A brief history of the term cellulite: In the1920s it was first heard in a France spa service area and then began to appear in publication in the 1960s Vogue magazine and now the world knows and uses the word cellulite in a Global scale.

Treatment – There are many, many topical creams and ointments that can be applied to the skin and there is collagenase injections treatment. Non-invasive procedures, there are mechanical message therapies, mechanical suction therapies, energy-based device such as radio frequency with deep penetration of the skin, ultrasound, laser, Coolsculpting, and other devices as well as surgical intervention that can be applied. Suggestion, stay with the non-invasive array. Please keep in mind that all procedures have an element of risk and that the risk factor greatly jumps higher when it comes to invasive attempts when injections and surgical intervention is used. Although I may go for the some of the non-invasive procedures, the surgical procedures are definitely out of my league. It is important to research, evaluate, talk to those that have had it done, talk to family members and friends before a decision is made especially with the more invasive procedures are being considered. What is written is extremely brief and not all the variations and methods are presented. Again, Research, Research, Research!

Surgical Fat Removal Techniques

Bariatric surgery is the minimization of food consumption by interfering with food adsorption in the intestinal tract.

Injection Lipolysis is an injection of a lipolyzing agent into the fat areas to be reduced.

Liposuction is a form of suctioning the fat cells from the human body in the attempt to change the shape of the body. The is the least effective method.

Cryolipolysis is a method of freezing the fat cells causing death to the fat cells

The typical cost for treatment or surgery depends on where you are going to have this done. In the U.S. the price range is from $750.00 to $1,500.00 and up.

Age and Fat Cells

As stated, the number of fat cells you have in your body have already been established and set early in infancy and childhood. By adolescence at the age of 20 the fat cells in young girls will double because of their hormones. Estrogen helps to increase the growth of fat cells and during post-pregnancy it reserves fat cells for breast feeding. In menopause, women start to mimic men's fat storage patterns. Through all this, fat cells in men and women will remain constant and it does not matter if you gain or loss weight. This constant fat cell number will even be there if you have liposuction, bariatric surgery, CoolSculpting, or any other form of fat cell surgical procedures to remove the cells. Your genetics will dictate and maintain the same body constant of fat cell number. You are the one that will determine your weight by what you put into your body. It is this that will determine the swelling of the adipocytes with lipids entering the fat cells which will expand the size of the fat cell. The amount of lipids in the fat cells and the numerous fat cells in the body is the causation of weight or an overweight condition and it is this that has to be controlled. As we age, losing weight does become more difficult due to the aging muscles and the slowing metabolism. This does not mean that you cannot shed and lose those excess fatty areas and yes, it will take more effort. Increasing muscle mass by resistance strength exercises and eating a balanced and nourishing diet will help equalize the metabolic changes in your body. Don't be afraid of adding high-protein foods to the list of foods like beans, lentils, nuts, and seeds. When it comes to stress, it is easy for one to tell you to reduce the stress but when your "up-tight" and your hormones secrete **cortisol** into the circulatory system that triggers the "fight or flight" response, it is not such an easy thing to control. Cortisol is a hormone that is stored in your fat cells and every time you become stressed-out unnecessarily or even with a good reason you can release this stored hormone in response to this stress and this you do not want to do. Activity such as exercise or a simple walk around the block will release some of this cortisol in a more controlled form. When you sleep, your body relaxes and the stresses, agitations, anger, and negative emotions are put aside. This would help your body and mind to recalibrate and refresh and to return back to a normal circadian rhythm. With less cortisol circulating the better you will feel. After all we have said about being overweight and how unhealthy it is, a question that is always in the air is "Can one be overweight and be health." This question is not entirely clear but researches say yes. To me, it all depends on the form and quality of life you have lived and how well you live this life depends on how well you continue this drive in the later part of your life journey. Is it a healthier form or a difficult, uncomfortable and painful form? This is what this book is all about, 'LIVING THE HEALTHIER FORM.

Chapter 11

The Law and the Elder Population

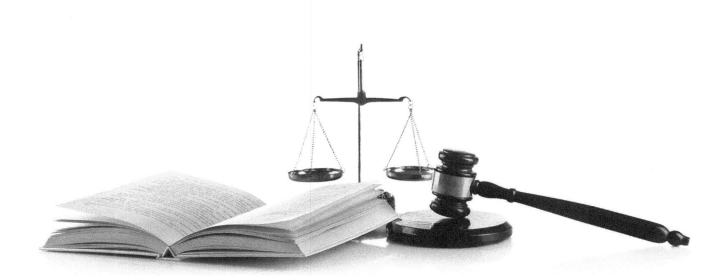

Contents in Chapter 11

The Law and the Older Population

There is something about the law that us non-lawyer types just do not understand. It seems that the law has its own language and yet there is some familiarity in the words and the phraseology of its meaning. Unlike medical terminology, chemical terminology or even scientific terminology; law seems, sounds, and is more understandable but just out of the normal range of clarity and comprehensibility for those of us that are not in the law profession. Albeit, it is not in any way like the technical verbiage of the scientific jargon which was just mentioned. The language of law is, in reality, regular English or better known as legal English using the more un-known phrases and words of the English language that would not normally be used in ordinary conversations. It is relegated to the area of reader-unfriendly or legalese. This makes it good for the practice of law but a pain in the butt for the rest of us. Please keep in mind that my intention is not to teach law or to provide a course in law but to give some referential information as to some of the fundament principles of law as it relates to the place it plays in our lives and more specifically in the lives of the elder and the law. Since elder law will pertain mostly with health care provisions of the law as it narrates to the health care professionals; it is important to learn some of their legal lingo. This chapter is intended and directed at the older person as a group and as an individual to help them navigate through some of the benefits and in the understanding of the legal initiatives of the rules of law in gerontology and geriatrics. This effort will entail a basic understanding of the rules of law and how it works, how it affects the older population, and the important influence it plays on the older population regarding the principle guidelines as we age. It will also be a valuable tool to you, your love ones, and to a wide spectrum of people that deal with and care for the elder population. Law is rather a complex subject so it is imperative to understand the essences of laws language by relaying a broad range of terms and phrases in the attempt, I hope, to simplify some of the legal jargons more appropriately.

Legal Systems and Elder Law

Legal needs for the older individuals have and still are a very challenging experience especially when it comes to the medical, social, and daily life activities (DLA) needs and other public and administrative care needs applicable to the elder population. They basically fall primarily under two facets of law:

1. **Medical jurisprudence** – The branch of law that deals with the application of law to medicine or, conversely, the application of medical science to legal problems. Medical

jurisprudence may be involved in cases concerning genetics relationships (paternity test) or injury or death resulting from violence. (From Elements of Jurisprudence by Theodric Romeyn Beck, M.D. – Vol. 1 Dec.11, 2018)

2. **Forensic medicine** – The application of medical knowledge to the investigation of a crime, particularly in establishing the cause of the injury or death.

Medical jurisprudence also covers informed consents, refusal of treatment, and termination of treatment as well as the legal aspects of confidentiality. When talking about forensics one thinks of criminal investigations and obtaining criminal evidence for criminal cases and procedures, well forensic medicine is basically the same. It tries to find course and effect in the medical arena to rule in or out any criminal causation of medical malpractice.

Elder laws have been enacted and government programs have been established primarily to help guide and care for the legal rights of the older population. These rights guide the elderly individuals and health caregivers care for the needs of the older population. Health care providers can range from family members, love ones, friends, or in the more professional area of health care the providers can be; physicians, nurses, pharmacies, and any and all allied health care professionals and practitioners. Understanding these laws as it pertains to the older population, though, can be difficult and confusing to interpret due to its impressive language **verbiage** (word usage). In order to overcome this selective legal mumbo-jumbo, one must try and learn a little of the legal terminology related to the law.

Law normally falls within four specific classifications; constitutional law, statutory law, administrative law, and common law.

Constitutional law is a body of laws that defines the roles, powers, and structures of the different entities within the state, that is, the executive, the parliament or legislature, and the judiciary which combines the basic rights of the citizens as it is related to the government.

Statutory law are laws written and passed by a body of legislators. Statutes may originate with national, state, or local legislatures in a municipality.

Administrative law is the body of law which regulates the operation and procedures governed by the rules, regulations, and orders of government agencies.

Common law is the part of English law that derived from customs and judicial precedents rather than statutes. This is often in contrast to statutory law. Common law is broken down into four types; criminal, civil, common, and statuate.

Government agencies are organized by the hierarchy or structure they hold over the land. The **federal government** is regulated by the United States Constitution, the overall authority that gives the power to tax the citizens which is used for the welfare of the citizens. These tax dollars are what pays for programs, such as, Medicare, interstate and foreign commerce, the

FDA, the FDCA, and many other services for the protection, health, and welfare of the people. The **state government** has a state Constitution that gives them authorization to control and regulate all affairs which include general welfare, health, and safety within the state. The state Constitution is inferior, in a legal sense, to the federal Constitution. Other powers are granted by the **"inherent parens patriae"** (parent of the fatherland) to protect all those unable to protect themselves. **Local governments** have the powers that are granted by laws that govern by the Constitution of the state in which they are a part of and in the same municipality or location. These laws continue down to the cities, counties, and other smaller municipalities. Each of the government branches follows the same general principles, processes, and procedures of the law as the **legislative branch** which is responsible for introducing laws, the **executive branch** to follow the laws as well as enforces the laws, the **judiciary branch** to interpret and regulate the constitutional laws and statutes and to provide insight into common law.

The Purpose of Law

There are many different meanings and definitions for the purpose of law but the simplest one is that it is a means to protect the people against those that wish to harm them. Law is the rule of conduct and action that has been prescribed by legal authority following principles that are readily understood by the average citizen. In fact, the first ten amendments and the fourteenth amendment to the Constitution of the United States of America specifically limits the federal and state governments from imposing or intruding on the rights of the citizens. It is a shield that grants certain privileges and rights to the citizens. After saying this, the government does have the right to set limits by law to controlling wrongful and harmful behavior, and has the authorization to enforce and punish those that violate these said laws. This process starts with those that do not respect the rule of law which is the bad action against the statutes of the law, such as, practicing medicine or nursing without a valid license, physicians not following government medical laws, their medical oath of medicine, Medicare rules and regulations and other entitled patient care acts. This bad action is then brought before the enforcement branch of the law where it is then brought before the people through the act of the courts. The case in court starts with the legal action of the **plaintiff** bringing a case against another in a court of law. This law action is against the person or **defendant** bringing a litigated or arraigned by the plaintiff. The defendant in a criminal case is also known as the **accused.** There are a number of ways to classify law but the simplest way is to say that law is divided broadly in to two general customs: **criminal law** and **civil law.**

A **civil law** is a **Tort law or common law** of civil wrong doing that causes a claimant to suffer loss or harm, that caused legal liability for the person who commits the tortious act. The punishment in tort cases is the monetary compensation that the court orders the defendant to pay the plaintiff. **Criminal law** (Penal Law) is a system of law concerned with the punishment of wrongful conduct in those that commit crimes. Criminal law and civil law have two venues of judicial procedure.

Criminal Law	**Civil Law**
Crimes as public wrong	Tort as private wrong
Punishment as incarceration or death	Punishment as compensation
Government as persecutor	Injured person as plaintiff
Proof: Beyond reasonable doubt	Proof: Preponderance of evidence

To break it down a little more there are a few legal terms and definitions one must get to know and understand.

- **Tort** – A wrongful act or conduct which gives rise to a civil suit.
- **Plaintiff** – A person who sues another.
- **Defendant** – A person/corporation/city agency being sued.
- **Negligence** – Is the occurrence when one improper action is taken or not taken or failure to take proper care in doing something.
- **Gross Negligence** – Intentionally harming of a person or patient. Acting with malice, intent or desire to injure or produce suffering in a person.
- **Reasonable man** – is a theory referring to the test whereby a hypothetical person is used as a legal standard, especially to determine if someone acted with negligence.
- **Abandonment** – The surrender, relinquishment, disclaimer or cessation of property or rights. Voluntary relinquishment of all rights titles, claims, and possessions, with the intent of not reclaiming it.
- **Health Care Proxy** – A patient identifies an agent permitted to make treatment decisions when the patient is no longer capable of such decision making. This is not honored in the pre-hospital setting. Used in the hospital only.
- **Living Will** – A statement of the patient's desires before he/she was incapacitated. This is not honored in the pre-hospital setting. Used in the hospital only.
- **Compensatory damages** – Are awarded to a plaintiff in a lawsuit as a way to repay them for the loss or harm they encountered as a result of a defendant's actions. They are intended to place the plaintiff in the position they would have occupied if not for the defendant's harmful act/s. It is also known as Actual damages.
- **Punitive damages** – is awarded for pain and suffering and is awarded where the conduct complaint merits punishment, hence the quantum, typically is larger and is added onto compensatory damages. It is also known as Exemplary damages.

Why Learn About Elder Law?

The aging population is growing rapidly and according to the U.S. Census Bureau taken in 2016, there are approximately 50,858,679 elder adults out of a total population of 325,719,178. Also taken from the U.S. Census Bureau is that this trend will continue to grow into the 2050's when the elder population can reach 88.5 million. The U.S. age population is continuing to grow older and people are living longer with the sidebar of having fewer children as well as a decrease in the younger population to maintain or sustain this growing movement. The racial diversity is also changing and there will be more females then men filling this population decrease. For the first time in history the older population in the U.S. will outnumber the children population by the year 2030 due to the decline in the number of births. Future long-term planning should be implemented for this varied change in population and a systematic approach should be established that will help this growing transformation inevitability modification. This includes new policies and funding's that should be allocated and geared towards elder care to prevent incidences with predators, perpetrators and elder abusers, and management issues such as risk factors, adults with disabilities, adults with dementia, and those in long term care facilities to mention just a few. Realizing that this should go without saying, I feel the urge to say it any way: No matter how old one is, justice and humanity requires that all people are equal and a full member of the society of human beings living in this world and should be treated with the respect and dignity that is bestowed to all humans of this community. These rights include those with disabilities be it physical or mental and all our efforts and capabilities should be to help and protect those that need our care. More on this later.

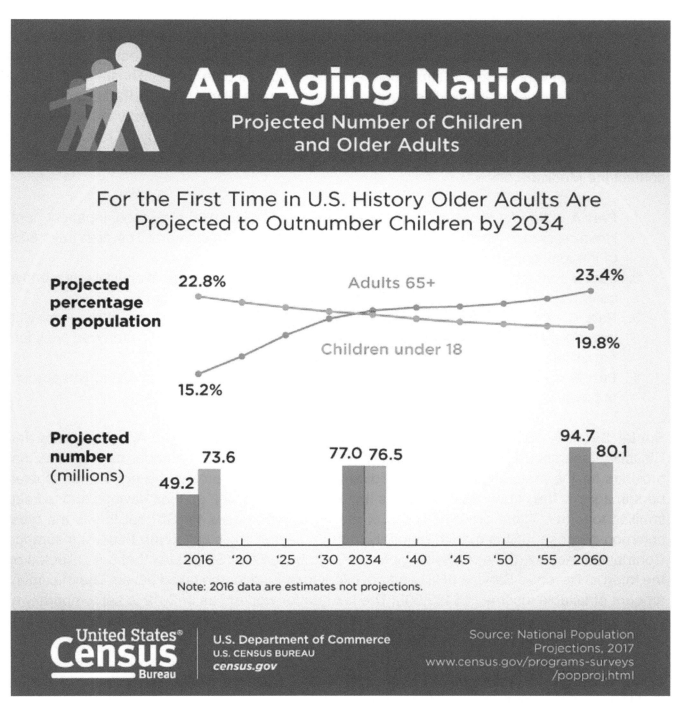

**An Aging Nation: Projected number of children and Older Adults (March 13, 2018).
From Census.gov>census Information and Visualization (Public Domain)**

Elder Care Help

There are many ways to get help and assistance for those that are in need of support. Many of these are government assistance programs and these support agencies are at the federal, state, and local levels. They can provide financial and healthcare requirements and other resources to senior citizens who need help.

Medicare is a federally funded program and its purpose is to provide basic health insurance to those age 65 and over, as well as to help other specifically qualified individuals. Medicare is not free; it is funded by the citizens of the United States through their payroll taxes. Medicare taxes are at 2.9% that was set in 2013 and they have no taxable income ceiling. These tax rates can change and are variable and flexible. It has a number of parts; Part A, Part B, Part C, and Part D and each Part provides a specific health service and/or coverage. The majority of beneficiaries choose Part A and Part B but Part B is not free and a small deduction may be required. There is so much to learn about the Medicare Benefit Plan that if this is what you feel you need then contact the Medicare office.

1. **Part A** is free for those who pay taxes and it covers hospital expenses, inpatient care, Hospice care, skilled nursing care, and limited home nursing care. The plan pays 80% of the total cost.
2. **Part B** cost about $104.90 each month as of 2015. It pays for physician visits, preventive care, check-ups, medical equipment and supplies in outpatient care.
3. **Part C** which is called Medicare Advantage is offered by Medicare through private insurance companies. It provides maintenance organizations, such as, preferred providers organization, and services for the special need's groups.
4. **Part D** is a prescription drug plan available through insurance companies. The amount of payment for the plan depends on the particular insurance company.

Social Security (SSI) is the commonly used term for the federal Old-Age, Survivors and Disability Insurance (OASDI). The act and related laws establish a number of programs that provides for the material needs of individuals and families; to protect the aged and disabled person against the expenses of illnesses that may otherwise use up their savings and to keep families together. There are other uses of the funding purposes for SSI but this is the most common purpose. SSI is funded primarily through payroll taxes called the Federal Insurance Contribution Act tax (FICA) or Self-Employed Contribution Act (SECA) tax that are collected by the Internal Revenue Service (IRS) and put into a trust fund for the taxed payee. The maximum amount of taxable income is $132,900. The tax rate for workers as of 2012 is set temporally at 4.2% while the employers rate remains at 6.2% giving 10.4% total rate. These tax rates can change and they are variable and flexible.

Administration on Aging (AOA) is an agency of the United States Department of Health and Human Services that works to try and maintain the independence of the older population within their communities. This is done by awarding grants to States, Native Americans tribal organizations, and local communities in the support of programs authorized by Congress in the Acts to Older Americans. This organization also supports research endeavors and projects that support these same goals. It ensures that these grants given are actively and progressively supporting, analyzing, and meeting the needs of an aging population. The AOA funds nutrition programs such as meals on wheels, ensuring that patients get to their doctors on time, buying groceries, and provides help that is given to caregivers. The website is **acl.gov/about-acl/administration-aging or acl.gov** then press the orange **I NEED HELP**

Department of Veterans Affairs (VA) provides complete healthcare benefits and services to military men and women at the veteran's hospital medical centers and outpatient clinics. The VA also provides non-healthcare benefits such as disability compensation, vocational rehabilitation, educational assistance, home loans, life insurance, and burial and memorial benefits to eligible veteran's and family members at 135 national cemeteries throughout the United States. The Veteran's Administration agency is overseen by the Secretary of Veteran's Affairs, a cabinet post that is appointed by the President with the consent and advice of the Senate. There are three main divisions and they are headed by the Undersecretary:

1. **Veteran's Health Administration (VHA)** is responsible for all health care in all its form.
2. **Veteran's Benefits Administration (VBA)** is responsible for registration eligibility determination, and key lines of business (benefits and entitlements):

   a. **Home Loan Guarantee**
   b. **Insurance**
   c. **Vocational Rehabilitation and Education**
   d. **Education (G.I. Bill)**
   e. **Compensation and Pension**

3. **National Cemetery Administration (NCA)** is responsible for providing burial and memorial benefits and maintenance of the VA cemeteries.

The Health Insurance Portability and Accountability Act (HIPAA) is a federal law enacted in 1996 that requires a national standard to protect sensitive patient health information from being disclosed without the patient's expressed consent or knowledge. This means that all patient health information is to be protected from fraud and theft and that addresses should be guarded and limited on health care insurance coverage. This federal law is called the **HIPAA Law.** If you feel that your health care information is being exposed, used, and/or leaked out the federal, state, local law enforcement authorities should be notified.

The Americans with Disabilities Act National Network (ADA) provides information, guidance, and training on how to implement assured equality of opportunity, full participation, independent living, and economic self-sufficiency for individuals with disabilities. There are 10 regional ADA National Networks located throughout the United States that can help. You can contact the ADA Center at 1-800-949-4232(vice).

The National Institutes of Health (NIH) is a primary agency of the U.S. Department of Health and Human Services (USNHHS) and the major purpose of the NIH is the responsibility for biomedical and public health research. It was formed in 1887 as part of the USDHHS and its purpose is to conduct scientific research through its Intramural Research Program (IRP) funding 1,200 principle investigators and more than 4,000 postdoctoral personal of which are non-NIH research members or facilities through this IRP funds. It funds research grants for heart disease, cancer, and strokes. NIH continues to research AIDS, women's health, and disease prevention. The National Institute on Aging is part of the NIH and it researches dementia and Alzheimer's disease. It will help in assessing, diagnosing, and managing all cognitive impairments. The NIH and the National Institute of Aging can be found on the website.

Your U.S. Senators, believe it or not, are one of the hardest agencies and/or people to contact in the United States. It's like, once they are elected by "THE PEOPLE" they fall into a vacuum only to be heard from on the radio, TV, or other media outlets. After saying that, your local Senator can be of great help to you in time of crisis in regard to building issues, health related concerns, financial needs, and many other needs and benefits not only for the elderly person but for the caregiver and love ones. Here are some ways of communicating with your local Senator:

Address
The Honorable (Name of Senator)
United States Senate
Washington, D.C. 20510

Correspondence to Senate Committee
Name of Committee – Senators Name
United States Senate
Washington, D.C. 20510

By telephone – U.S. Capital Switchboard at 202-224-3121

Your Congressional Representatives goes into this same void once elected but there are more Congressional Representatives then Senators in each state. At this time, in 2020, there are 27 Representatives in New York State which means that currently NYS comprises 27 districts and each district elects one Congressional Representative. New Jersey has 12 Congressional districts with 12 Representatives. It should be easier to communicate with them then a Senator of which ALL states just have but two. Both can be of great help and of great benefit to you for all the same reasons.

Address
The Honorable (Name)
House Office Building
U.S. House of Representative
Washington, D.C. 20515

President of the United States
The White House
President (Name)
1600 Pennsylvania Avenue N.W.
Washing, D.C. 20500

There is a Comment Line: 202-456-1111 and a Fax Line 202-456-2461 and an Email line to the President which is whitehouse.gov. You can communicate to any White House Staff member through the Comment Line and the Fax Line.

Medicaid serves is the nation's primary source of health insurance coverage for low-income population in the United States. Each State sets their own Medicaid program eligibility standards, determinations, and sets the rate of payment for this aid. The rate of payments varies from State to State and because one qualifies in one State does not mean that person will be eligible in another State. The State does not have to participate in the Federal Medicaid funded program. The Federal Government has a strict poverty line that does vary with individuals and families as well as families with dependent children. There are different agencies within the Medicaid program and jointly the Federal Government will finance seniors and fund medical expenses as it will with all ages and will pay nearly all of the long-term care cost. For any of these programs, you can also access help and assistance by using your website. There are two websites that can help you and your love one/s obtain the support needed and the assistance to find out what programs you and your love one/s need and are eligible for as well as many other programs within your community that might be of continuous service.

- ✓ **www.Benefits.gov:** – Is a benefit finder for elder assistance and it ranges from the federal, state, and local agencies. The needs of your love one/s should be gathered and all the necessary information needed should be carefully reviewed such as their state of health, disability, income, assets, military service, educational level, and any other valuable information before accessing this site. In this Benefits Finder, there will be an on-line form/s to be completed so it is important to have all this information correctly available for input on the site. Once you have submitted the questionnaire, a list of government programs, supplements, and services information on how to apply to these services will be sent to you.
- ✓ **www.Benefitscheckup.org** – This site is run by the non-profit National Council on Aging that was developed for the senior citizens. They will ask for the same questions and information as Benefits.gov: but it will have more programs for the elder population.

What is good about these programs is that it gives free senior care guides, practical tips, and expert advice to help your aging love one/s to include Family care for the family, Finding and Managing Home Care, Alzheimer's and Dementia Care, Guide to Veteran's Benefits, Funeral Planning Guide, and much more information. Other organizations and agencies that will guide and assist senior citizens are:

1) **The AARP Foundation**
2) **AARP Caregiver Support – Caregiver at Home**
3) **Caregiver for Seniors – care.com Official Site**
4) **How to get Government Assistance for Elders: 12 Steps**
5) **Government Programs and Benefits for Seniors/Senior Care Homes**
6) **NYC Department of the Aging**

Before sending information to the non-government organizations, it is strongly advised to review what it is that they are offering and if it really fits into your love one's needs and how it helps in the long run of care.

Other Countries Health Care System

Just of an informational and educational interest, Canada's healthcare system is delivered to the people and funded by the people of Canada through the provincial and territorial system of the public taxes. This system was started in Canada around1984 and it is called the universal Canada Health Act. Tommy Douglas introduced this plan while serving his tenure as Premier of Saskatchewan. Healthcare in Canada is funded and administered by the 13 provinces and territories and the guidelines and standards are set by the Canadian Federal Government to ensure that a consistence level of care is established across the country. As states, it is funded through taxation, as well as, public funding to Canadians at no expense or out-of-pocket-cost. This healthcare services covers all medical costs, needed medications, vaccinations, etc. Each province may not have the same program but still most follow the federal governments guidelines in providing services. In Great Britain, their healthcare system is state funded and is called the National Health Service (NHS) which guarantees healthcare to all its citizens. It provides healthcare coverage without out-of-pocket-cost to the needed individuals. Both Canada and Great Britain do accept private health insurance companies' insurances plans from other countries.

When traveling or vacationing to other countries, it is a wise investment decision to check on that countries healthcare system, including their EMS response system and emergency service, medication availability requirements, emergency transportation availability back to your country of origin, and accepted insurance coverage. The Department of Health should also be called to find out if there are any health issues to worry about in the country you are visiting.

Elder Rights

It seems rather strange that there are separate and specific laws to protect our senior citizens yet according to the **National Council on Aging (NCOA),** it is believed that the elder population are one of the highest abused population of all age groups. Approximately 1 in 10 Americans age 60+ have experienced some form of elder abuse. When you use that statistics, the range of elder abuse is as high as 5 million each year. These are just the reported cases of abuse which in actuality the range can fluctuate up or down accordingly. These abusers are from elder men and women and can be from love-ones such as family members with the majority of the perpetrators being the adult children and spouse of the abused victim, so says the **NCOA (ncoa.org).** Again, using the NCOA statistics and assessing what makes the older population such easy targets is that in some cases their cognitive mental acuteness is impaired or are to physically fragile to respond. Another reason which makes them so venerable is that they not have very many social friends which makes them socially isolated. Those that have a form of dementia have experienced the highest of this disrespectful, abusive, and neglectful behavior. This type of abuse also extends to those that have different forms of physical disabilities. Elder abuse does not only mean by neglecting the health and welfare of the older adult; it can also mean an assault-battery and wrongful touch, sexual abuse, and even verbal abuse. Naming some elder abuses are:

- **Physical abuse** is when physical force is used intentionally to harm the senior. This can include any non-accidental use of force to the senior resulting in physical pain, injury, or impairment.
- **Psychological abuse** is any action that causes emotional distress to the senior. This can take the form of intimidation, humiliation and ridicule, and habitual blaming and scapegoating. Other emotional abuses are ignoring the senior, isolating the senior from friends, terrorizing and menacing the senior.
- **Sexual Abuse** is the forcible act of a sexual nature against an elder person will and/or the senior not being able to give consent due to a psychological condition such as dementia or Alzheimer's disease.
- **Financial Abuse** is the unauthorized use of a senior's funds or property without the senior's prior permission. This can involve a caregiver or an outside scam artist. Financial exploitation and scam artist target the elder daily such as "prizes" the elder won but must pay to obtain, fake charities, and investment fraud. Be careful with doctors and nurses as well as hospital charges.
- **Neglect abuse** is when a caregiver does not attend to the senior's needs. Example: not giving them enough food or water, not helping them to wash up or bathe, leaving them alone and unattended.
- **Self-abuse** is when the elder stops taking care of their own needs. This is noticeable with bad personal hygiene, letting their surroundings become dirty, not paying their bills, and not drinking or eating enough food.

If you suspect that your love one is being abused in any way call the Adult Protective Services. If you feel that your love one is in immediate danger call the nearest police department and/ or 911. The problem with elder abuse is that there are many warning signs of abuse such as bruises, abrasions, burns, and more obvious signs like pressure made by bedsores, and broken bones. Check for any sudden changes in emotional, alertness, unusual depression, frequent arguments with caregiver or other adults. Do you hear or see any emotional abuse like belittling remarks or threats, abuse of power and over controlling by patient or caregiver? Some of the best ways in preventing elder abuse is educating yourself of the laws, knowing your professionals and caregivers, staying publicly active, and knowing your rights as an advocate for senior citizens. Other ways are by staying socially active with friends, maintaining your health by visiting your doctor routinely, checking your Will periodically, and just be alert and responsive to your surroundings. If you are an advocate for your love one/s, visit them frequently and look in their refrigerate, check out the home are apartment for cleanliness, and use all your olfactory senses for signs of disarray and unsafe conditions. This goes for those in nursing homes also.

Legal Preparation for the Elderly

Although this heading is "Legal Preparation for the Elderly" it really should read "Life Preparations for All." This section will briefly cover Wills, Living Wills, Power of Attorney, and other preparatory elements that should be foreseen during this journey through life. One always must keep in mind that; in many circles it is taboo to talk Wills or about getting old or dying but barring a tragic accident all of us will eventually become older.

Will and Testament

A Will is a legal document in which a person expresses their wish as to how their property is to be distributed upon the death of the testator or person who made out the Will or given legacy. The Will names an **executor** to manage the estate until it is finally distributed. A Will may also create a testamentary or trust that is only effective after the death of the testator. The term **Will** is a valid legal document that applies to both personal and real property. The requirements for writing a Will is any person over the age of majority and being of sound mind can write or make a Will. The title of the document should read **"Last Will and Testament"** on the face of the document. A **codicil** or statement that you hereby revoke all previous Wills and other codicils should be made. The Will must be signed and dated in the presence of two or more disinterested witnesses (check with your state). Your signature must be placed at the end of the Will. Anything in writing after your signature will be ignored. Although there is no legal requirement for you to seek out a lawyer to write your Will, it is strongly advised that you do because there are many ways that self-written Wills can fail in a challenge in a court of law. Just for added knowledge, there are a number of different types of Wills:

- **Nuncupative (non-culpatory)** is an orally dictated Will that is often limited to sailors or military personal.

- **Holographic Will** are Wills written in the hand of the person writing the Will or testator. In many jurisdictions, the signature and the material terms of the holographic Will must be written only in the hands of the testator.

- **Self-prove Will** is a Will that comes with something extra: a sworn statement from the witness who watched the Will-maker sign the Will. In many states, the probate court will accept this Will as a statement of evidence that the Will is valid.

- **Notarial Will** is a way of limiting the chances that someone will contest your Will wishes. A notarial Will is a kind of formal Will drawn up by a notary republic and requires the presence of a witness or in certain cases two witnesses. Problems do come when the Will is drawn up by the testator.

- **Mystical Will** is a Will that at this time is only applicable in Louisiana and is a Will that is prepared and signed in secret. It is also known as a Secret Will, Closed Will, or Sealed Will.

- **Reciprocal/mirror/mutual/husband and wife Wills** are sometimes used by married couples as a simple means of securing the transfer of property to the other spouse upon their death.

- **Serviceman's Will** is a Will of a person in active military service and usually lacking certain formalities, particularly under English law.

- **Unsolemn Will** is a Will in which the executor is unnamed.

- **Will in solemn form** is a form of probate of a Will where the Will is decreed in open court to be the Last Will and Testament after notice to all interested persons and after the testimony of the attesting witness.

There are things that one should understand when writing a Will. This is important especially if you have land and property to share, a store or other estates to petition out. Do you want to have a **beneficiary,** how many and what percentage to each and/or do you want to bequeath a gift or property? Who will be your executor or person to **administer** the estate and a person who has the duty under the Wills trust to ensure that the right beneficiaries in the Will are upheld? Wills are not an easy instrument to write and should be thought out very carefully before, during, and after visiting an attorney. Again, Wills can be changed and once done should be reviewed frequently.

Living Wills

It is commonly believed that a Living Will and other advance directives are just for the elderly population to worry about. This is very far from the truth. Life is a mystery and everyday a new beginning which really means that anything can happen unexpectedly, out of the blue at any age. As an adult, there is no waiting time for the unexpected to happen that is why it is important to prepare these documents now. Living Wills are written legal documents that is prepared beforehand given instructions when one is unable to make these decisions. It is this planning ahead for life's unexpected medical care and for one to avoid unnecessary suffering during times of emergency situations. It gives you a voice when you're unable to and reduces confusion or disagreements about how you want to be treated and cared for during this crisis in time. It spells out the concept and expectation of the medical treatment you would want in keeping you alive. Do you want all the treatment available to extend your life on all situations or is there a situation where you do not want all life saving measures? If there is a cure soon to be discovered, do you want treatment for the eventuality that that cure will be of help? It is up to you to determine the situation and the possible end-of-life decision in your Living Will. Discuss this with family and your doctor about these medical decisions:

- **Cardiopulmonary resuscitation (CPR)** is when your heart stops beating and your desire to have CPR done or not done. Do you want a defibrillator (electric shock) used to stimulate the heart?
- **Mechanical ventilation** is a device to help you to breath. Do you want a breathing device to take over your breathing if breathing becomes a problem: if yes when and how long do you want it to be used?
- **Tube feeding** is a means of force feeding the body with nutrients and fluids either intravenously or via a tube in the stomach. You can choose one or all methods and how long you want this method to continue.
- **Dialysis treatment** if your kidney fails. Do you want dialysis help to remove waste from your blood stream and helps balance fluids levels in the body?
- **Antibiotics or antiviral medication** to treat infections. Determine if you want the infections to be treated aggressively or allow the infection to run its course.
- **Comfort care (palliative care)** is any intervention to keep and manage pain and make one comfortable until all wishes are met. You must specify to what extent and for how long.
- **Organ and tissue donations** can be written in your Living Will.
- **Donating your body for scientific studies** can also be specified in your Living Will.

Do not resuscitate (DNR) or **do not intubate (DNI)** does not have to be in your Living Will, you just need to tell your doctor and He or She will write it in the orders and put them in your medical records. Be safe and write them in your Living Will any way. It is a good idea to inform the hospital staff about your DNR and DNI concerns each time you are admitted into the hospital or healthcare facility.

Power of Attorney

This is a person that you have given medical and/or healthcare authority in making decisions for you when you are not able to do so for yourself. It is also called **durable power of attorney** and there are other names depending on where you live in the U.S. for this healthcare proxy. It is very important to wisely choose an agent as your healthcare proxy because some situations may require good judgement. This requires a mature knowledgeable person that is able to and willing to make decisions and discuss medical care with your medical provider. One that can be trusted to stay with your values and desires and is able to advocate for you if there is a disagreement about your care. This person can be a family member such as your spouse or other member of the family, a friend, and even a person from your religious order. It is important to choose more than one person to fulfill this important role.

Once these documents are completed, make sure that your doctor is aware of these forms and that you gave a copy to your lawyer and all those that you have informed of regarding your Living Will, as well as, your healthcare agent and any other healthcare provider. Let the important people in your life know about the advance directives and talk to them about your choices and decisions. Miniaturize a wallet-size copy of the healthcare forms that have your advance directives and keep it with you wherever you go. You can make changes to your advance directives at any time and this will require making out a new form and distributing them as before.

Case Study

I have a scenario for you to ponder. It is one of the reasons that I have decided to learn and understand more about who I am and where it is that life is eventually going to take me. It is also important and very enlightening to know how others envision and see older adults as the aging process takes its toll on this remarkable form of God's creative inspiration. Look this case over and see if there is any reason to think that this older adult was treated well or discriminated against because of his age.

A 75-year-old Hispanic man is getting into his parked car when a tractor with a 54-foot trailer passes him on the left side. The tractor is making a left hand turn on a narrow street and as the tractor makes this left turn the back end of the trailer weaves to the right crushing his left hand and fingers of this 75-year-old man against the open edge of his car door with the back end of the trailer. The old man's second, third, and fourth fingers are crushed with the fourth finger of the left hand having the top part of the finger severed completely off. This was witnessed by a number of pedestrians; one person, in her car, chased down the driver of the tractor trailer to stop him and inform him what has happened and another witness came to the aide of the accident victim. It is at this time that it was noticed that part of the fourth finger was missing and the injured pedestrian and the witness went back to the scene of the accident and found the severed finger. The witness went into the nearby store to get ice and a plastic bag and put the severed part of the finger into the bag with the ice. Other witnesses had already made calls to 911 and within five minutes the police and ambulance arrived. The patient's hand was dressed and treated by the EMT's and after a short debate as to the closest hospital to go to that had an orthopedic surgical team the ambulance took off and in approximately 7 minutes the patient was in the emergency room being prepped for surgery.

Within less than an hour of this old man's arrival, a short male walked into the patient's emergency room cubical and the patient assumed that this was a doctor. For this scenario we'll just say that he was a doctor. This person or doctor was in a white doctor's gown and just looked at the 75-year-old patient laying in the bed with I.V.'s in his arms and bandages around his left hand. He just stared at the patient and made no remarks or announcements. He does not announce who he is or give a name. On the right side of this doctor there is an Asian female dressed in a white doctors' gown and on his left, there is a blonde Caucasian female dressed exactly the same way. The patient thought that they may be two of the doctor's medical assistance. All three walked up to the bed of this 75-year-old man lying on the stretcher. This doctor continued to stare at the old man and the old man stares back meeting him eye to eye for what seems like minutes but was probably seconds. The doctor finely says "We have decided not to reattach the missing part of the finger. It looks too damaged." The doctor and his colleagues then turn around and walked out of the cubicle area and out of the emergency room. Approximately 45 minutes later, a nurse comes over and tells the patient that he will be transported to another affiliating hospital to see another orthopedic specialist and that surgery to his hand will be done there. The patient is put on another stretcher, re-packaged for transport and wheeled out of the emergency room to a waiting ambulance. Within 10 minutes the ambulance arrives at another hospital emergency room. From the emergency room he is taken to the operating room and is prepped for surgery again. Within 15 minutes another doctor walks into his cubical area where the 75-year-old Hispanic patient is and tells the patient his name and that he is the surgeon that would be performing the surgery. He then tells the patient "As you already know, the severed part of the fourth finger will not be reattached. The third finger is so badly damaged that there is a possibility that it cannot be repaired or saved. I will do my very best to try and save the finger." This surgeon then went out to the waiting room area and spoke to the patient's family regarding the surgical procedure. A few minutes later the patient was transported into the surgical suite. The surgeon was successful in saving the third finger. The question you are asked to answer is; was this the type of treatment you would want your love-one to receive and is this how you think he should be treated and cared for in both hospitals? Yes or No

Chapter 12

Falls and Accidents of the Elder Population

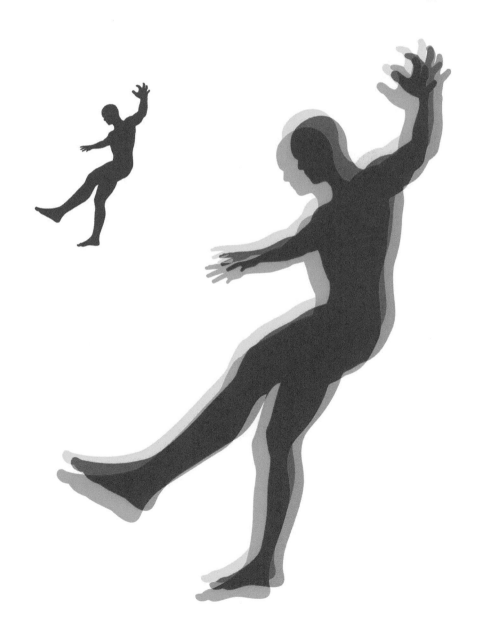

Contents in Chapter 12

Falls and Accidents of the Elder Population

Falls are one of the leading causes of injuries and deaths to senior citizens and the one factor that threatens their independence. Falls are not respectively directed only to the older population. Falls are going to happen even in those that age normally and in all age groups; the fact is, as we age our physiological and cognitive functions are also aging and according to the U.S. Center for Disease Control and Prevention in collaboration with National Council on Aging and I quote:

1) One in four Americans age 65 and over will sustain a fall each year.
2) Every 11 seconds, an older adult is treated in the emergency room for a fall; every 19 minutes, an older adult will die from a fall.
3) Falls are the leading cause of injuries and the most common cause of nonfatal trauma-related hospital admissions among older adults.
4) Falls result in more than 2.8 million injuries treated in the emergency departments annually, including over 800,000 hospitalizations and more than 27,000 deaths.
5) In 2015, the total cost of fall injuries was $50 billion. Medicare and Medicaid shouldered 75% of these costs.
6) Falls financial toll for the older adult is expected to increase as the population of older Americans grow and may reach as high as $67.7 billion by 2020.

Since the information above was deduced in 2015 and it is now 2020, it is believed that we have already reached this $67.7 billion threshold and the trend is just going to go higher. This statistics of injuries and mortality rate when it comes to falls extends to both sexes and to all racial and ethnic groups. Many times, these falls start even sooner as the age increases around 30 and 40 when the body's equilibrium and muscle tone starts to change and so the increase in the falls potentiality rises: frailty, poor vision, cochlea problems, postural imbalance, ambulatory disability, poor health, and declining overall biological functions can all contribute to this state of potential falls. Other risk factors of falls are medication use, psychological and/or physical impairment all are added possibilities of sensory deficits. It is said that seniors 70 and over have the highest potential of falls such as slipping on a wet surface, on an unsecured rug, in the snow or ice can all lead to very serious injuries. There is a set of opinions and agreements that most falls occur in the home/apartment as to what specific area in the home or apartment is still not clear. As to the gender, more men fall in the garage or on a walkway around the home and as of the data obtained in 1997-1998 from the **National Health Interview Survey (NHIS)** women are more likely to fall in the home. Statistically, the NHIS states that 55% of all fall injuries occurred in the home, 23% outside near the home, and only 22% of elder adults falls occurred away from the home. I do not know what you think of this but I find this to be pretty amazing. The safest place, our home, is the place where the most falls happen! The negative effect of how aging and its senescence influences our health's outcome has been well outlined above and studied through research by many organizations in the past and this study will continue into the future. The majority of these studies are based on studying the frail adult, and those that have risk factors such as preexisting medical conditions and disabilities but is this the only ones that fall or is there other underlining circumstances that predispose older adults to falls?

Why do Older People Fall?

The question is, are falls only a senior problem and due to age alone? Using this as a basis for our judgement on age only or on poor reflexes or tripping we should reexamine and reanalyze some facts. While medications do have side effects and health conditions are contributing factors in falls and the majority of falls in the home are due to "simple slips and trips" that are not directly due to any risk factor but just an unsafe home, I think falls can and will happen to all age groups. In fact, according to **"The Lancet"** Article/volume 381, issue 9860, P47-54 January 05, 2013, by Simon Fraser University and analyzed by Robinovitch's team and released in 2012 to The Lancet, most falls occurred from incorrect weight shifting, trips and stumbling, hits or bumps, loss of support, and collapses. These happen while forward walking, standing quietly, and sitting down. In their interpretation – "By providing insight into the sequences of events that most commonly lead to falls, our results should lead to more valid and effective approaches for balance assessment in all falls with a special eye on fall prevention in frail and those with risk factors that need long-term care." Although this information is valuable as stated, there is still this negative effect for those that do have risk factors and/or physical disabilities. Not disputing this assessment on falls, there is an additional aspect that must be considered and that is the emotional trauma to the fall victim and the staggering financial cost to the patient and the health care system as stated previously.

Medical Debts

Before we discuss safety and preventative fall measures, it would be a good idea to go over medical debts and cost of a sudden and unexpected hospital expense from a fall or an illness. This is what worries most seniors on a fixed income and what can cause or contribute to bankruptcy according to the American Journal of Public Health in 2019. This is the biggest problem faced by the senior citizen population in America. There are ways to navigate around some of the financial burden of hospital cost. That is not to say that you will escape all payments but it will help in some of the cost or give you more time to pay. According to the AARP Bulletin, December 2019, Vol. 60 No. 10:

1. Hospitals and doctors do not charge interest and they do not charge late fees as most other debtors do. This will give you more time to find or secure the necessary finance. This debt will go on credit score reports but once paid this will be removed from your report.

2. Asking the hospital or the doctor to help you reduce your payment is another way. Most hospitals have charity care and financial assistance policies for the needy and low-income people especially your nonprofit hospitals and those under IRS rules. Even the for-profit hospitals have some form of financial assistance but these hospitals can shape the polices for this financial assistance that will help with finance.

3. Low-income patients may qualify for Medicaid assistance. This assistance may pay for retroactive coverage of bills. It is advised that you do not take out a home equity loan or reverse mortgage for this would put your home at risk so says Jennifer Bosco a staff attorney at the National Consumer Law Center. She continues to say that it doesn't make sense to put medical bills on a credit card because you lose the ability to negotiate with your doctor.

4. If this debt is not payed or there is no good faith attempt of payment, the hospital/doctor have the right to forward this debt to the debt collectors who will take over the collection of this debt. Now it comes under the federal Fair Debt Collection Practice Act (FDCPA) and this act controls the manner and method of collection. This means that they cannot threaten or intentionally annoy you with phone calls, harass, oppress or abuse you and they must stop contacting you if you ask them. They do have the right to bring you to court for the collection of the debt and if they win, they can garnish your wages although Social Security and VA benefits cannot be garnished and are protected.

5. Do not assume that all collector debts are correct regarding your medical debt. You have 30 days from the day you are informed to ask questions and ask for proof regarding the amount you supposedly owe. Until this debt is validated, all collectors' efforts must seize until clarified.

I cannot stress the important and value of being a member of AARP and how it can help all of us mature senior adults and guide us through these trying times.

Getting to the hospital may be more of a problem then one may think. As stated, 55% of all fall injuries occur at home/apartment or near their home and in most cases while the older person is by themself. The problem is how to communicate to others and how would this elder accident victim summon emergency help if the injury is one that has incapacitated the injured person's ability to talk and/or walk. This scenario has happened on many occasions at home or in the garden. There are two medical alert systems one can rent although they can be pricey; **Medical Alert** and **Mobile Help.** These systems have automatic fall detection systems and the Mobile Help will go wherever you go and will allow you to be more independent, Medical Alert will only work in the home or apartment. To add to this, it is a good idea to carry in your wallet or purse a list of medications you're taking with the time and frequency of administrations especially diabetes, epilepsy, hypertensive, and mood stabilizer medications. You can also buy a wrist bracelet, necklace, and ankle bracelet with these medications listed. These are just smart things to do and good choice to make. More on this later.

Cause and Effect of Elder Falls

Much of what is going to be said has been said earlier but it is worth repeating time and again. It is important to understand that even the older people that are strong and have some risk factors or those that do have risk factors fall just like the young active people can. Age poses its own added problems to the equation and adding a sedentary lifestyle as a multiplier will increase this risk aspect substantially. You see, the natural aging process itself can contribute to an increase in fall potential. This normal aging process can affect vision or hearing and this alone can make you more venerable and likely to fall. When you add an illness or physical condition to this assessment both can syphon needed energy and strength away and increase an imbalance state. An unsafe home/apartment is just as dangerous as all medical conditions combined, such as, rugs not secured to the floor, poor lighting system in the home, wobbly chairs or tables, shaky banisters on the stairs, scattered clothing and shoes on the floor, to mention a few. Now you add the side effects of medication even some over-the-counter medication (OTC) can make one drowsy, sleepy or dizzy. Taking two or more medications or OTC and a prescription medication together may also be a contributing factor to falls. If you are taking certain herbal ingredients in combination with other essential drugs, OTC or prescribed, this total administration may be a dangerous mixture and you should consult a doctor for advice. To categorize some safety tips a little better;

- ✓ Wet or recently polished floors especially in the bathroom and kitchen areas,
- ✓ Dimly lit places like hallways, rooms, and walk areas,
- ✓ Rugs and carpets that are not secured to the floor,
- ✓ Reaching high or low in areas such as kitchen cabinets, storage areas, and closets,
- ✓ Stairways that are poorly lite and/or cluttered,
- ✓ Using OTC medications be it herbal, allergy, or pain relief medication,
- ✓ Combining OTC medications with prescription medications.

These are all potential accidents ready to happen. Ask about some of the main reasons you are taking these medications and ask your doctor about the possible side effects of your medication and fall potentials as well as other untoward affects and health conditions. Your healthcare provider should also be aware of the fall potentials that medications and physical environment conditions may potentiate especially medical situations of their patient, such as;

- **Chronic health conditions,** such as, heart disease, diabetes, dementia, and hypertension which can cause dizziness,
- **Impairments,** such as, poor vision, muscle wasting or weakness,
- **Illnesses** that can affect balance, such as, labyrinthitis (inflammation of the inner ear and cochlea).

Before discussing preventative measures in avoiding falls, I think it is a good idea to discuss what is an equilibrium disfunction. As we have stated, most falls occur when we are standing or sitting trying to move our body to rapidly or turning our heads too quickly. These balance disorders can be a disturbance with the labyrinth or vestibule area within the ear that informs the brain of the body's position in time, space, and place as well as it controls the positioning and movement of the head. The eye also sends positioning information to the brain and if one of them are faulty or does not match the labyrinth positioning in the ear, the brain has problems trying to interpret which is the actual position of the head in comparison to the body and imbalance occurs. There are three imbalance disorders to understand, dizziness, vertigo, and imbalance.

Dizziness is an altered sense of balance and is described as lightheadedness, feeling faint, as if your head is swimming and floating. Example: motion sickness symptoms and dizziness, nausea, and vomiting can occur.

Vertigo is a very specific kind of dizziness as if everything is going around and around in a circle; this can suddenly happen for internal or external reasons. This spinning sensation can be triggered by moving one's head or getting out of bed too fast or walking too quickly even looking up at the sky or tall buildings.

Imbalance can be caused by just walking and performing normal every day events. This can be the result of inner ear complications. Abnormalities in the ear can cause a sensation of floating or heavy head and unsteadiness.

Some of the other causes are; ear infection, head injury, circulatory problems, medications, and low or high blood pressure to name a few.

Preventing Falls

No one can prevent all falls so lets state that now. We can prevent the falls that are from carelessness, unsafe conditions, and those that you having the knowledge and the forethought to observe to be unsafety. There are obvious ways to stay safe and prevent falls but some are not so straight forward, for instance, I see a lot of females wearing toe slippers (flip-flops) or this type of slipper footwear in the streets. This is an accident ready to happen. Wear shoes and footwear that control the ankles and are secured to the feet with nonskid soles and at home use full formed slippers and not clogs, better yet, go bare foot. Make sure there are night lights in all dark areas of the home and remove all rugs that are not secured to the floor. In the bathroom, put grab bars for assistance in the toilet area and bath area and do not wax the floors at all not even with nonskid wax. I have illustrations of some safer shoes to wear. Now I'm going to mention the obvious things to help maintain good balance:

1. Exercise regularly, especially walking. Do more exercises in a standing position.
2. When exercising work the muscles that you use for walking and lifting.
3. Do not smoke.
4. Sleep is important to recalibrate the brain.
5. A good diet to nourish the brain.
6. Alcohol should be limited to two drinks a day or less.
7. See your doctor yearly for a physical exam and have your eyes and hearing checked and follow his/her advice on treatments and recommendations.

Your family can help make your home a safe haven and they can help determine the safety of your walk, gait and the steadiness on standing and sitting. Your doctor will also assess other parameters. Do not hesitate to call your family or your doctor in the event medical need arise.

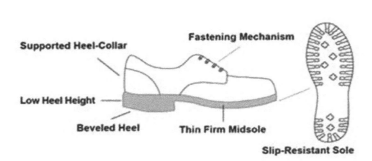

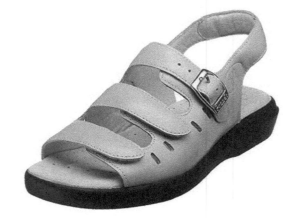

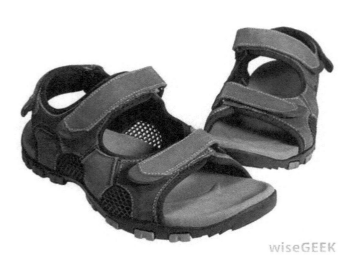

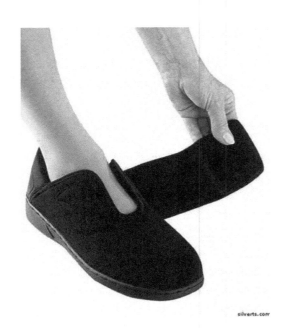

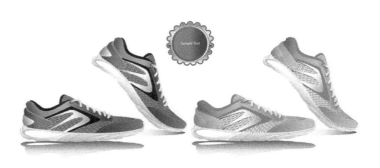

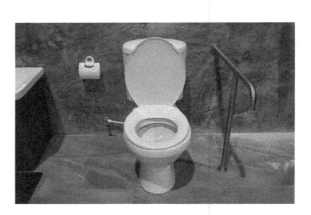

Sneakers are a very firm support for the feet

Toilet grab bar

Falls and Injury Risk Assessments

I dear say that many of these adverse health care outcomes when it comes to falls and the resulting injuries typically strike those over the age of 85 years, the fact is that many of these falls can be prevented. As time marches on and the old become older one can understand how statistically the incidences of falls and the increase in more serious injuries continue to rise. Although some facts have been covered, there are basic underlining factors that must be understood in more detail as to what contributes to the more serious injuries related to the fall potential:

Physical condition of the older adult at the time of the fall, any history of previous falls, are there orthopedic concerns such as osteoporosis, osteopenia, is there any numbness of the legs or other neuropathies in the limbs, has the senior had a bone density test and does he/she have a history of bone density problems or previous history of fracture.

Medications can alter judgement, balance, and mood. Medications can reduce reflex and cause slower movements and balance impairment as well as vision disturbances and slow wittedness of responses to positioning and movement can follow.

Cognitive decision-making abilities can be impaired due to dementia, delirium, Parkinson's disease, and slow wittedness due to stroke, trauma, alcohol or drugs. Nutritional deficiency such as B12 and diabetes can all cause cognitive impairment.

Functional ability of judgement can be a factor, that is, agitation or over estimation of the situation and decision, such as, speed, distance, and equalizing-positioning of objects in space and time can develop.

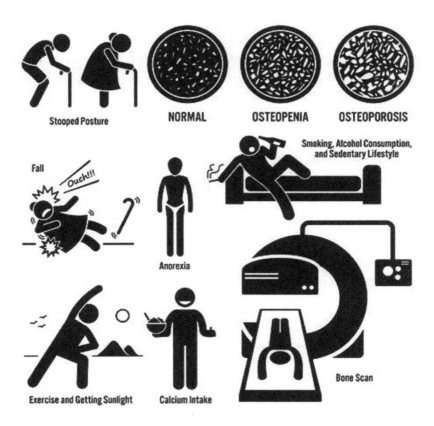

Stooped Posture — NORMAL — OSTEOPENIA — OSTEOPOROSIS

Fall — Ouch!!! — Anorexia — Smoking, Alcohol Consumption, and Sedentary Lifestyle — Bone Scan

Exercise and Getting Sunlight — Calcium Intake

As you can see falls will happen but safety prevention of falls due to unnecessary and neglectful conditions can be stopped and fall accidents reduced. We have covered the physiological and psychological risk aspects in falls such as visual problems, walking problems, depression, cognitive impairment, mobility deficit (stability), etc.; these are called **"intrinsic risk factor."** We have covered the environmental aspects of falls such as slippery rugs, bathrooms lacking grab rails, and slippery floor surfaces, etc.; these are called **"extrinsic risk factors"** aspects. Now, it is time to deal with the patient. One of the most prevalent senior concerns should be "is the patient eating and drinking enough on a daily basis." Nutrition is the key for muscle nourishment and for proper function. Without proper sustenance the muscles, organs, and nervous systems will just waste away. If the older adult does not drink adequate fluids for daily hydration, dehydration will occur. This can and has happened to many older adults. Other reasons such as diarrhea, excessive sweating, loss of blood, high temperature, diseases such as diabetes and the side effects of medications like diuretics can be primary or secondary considerations. Signs and symptoms of dehydration in seniors may include: confusion, walking difficulty, headaches and dizziness, dry mouth, sunken eyes, the inability to perspire or produce tears, rapid heart rate, and low blood pressure to mention a few. The concern of drinking 8 glasses of water a day is not totally true because it varies from person to person. This fluid intake does not only have to come from drinking water. Much of the fluids we take in comes from the foods we eat. Albeit it, this idea that coffee or tea beverages which has caffeine will dehydrate an older adult is not completely true. There is more water in coffee and in tea beverages than caffeine so it will still be a good way to hydrate the elder person. This goes for beer also but there is a point when the diuretic effects of caffeine and alcohol will kick in, so the key is moderation.

It seems like it always comes down to you, does it not. You have to keep yourself physically active. Take a portion of time out of a 24-hour day to exercise. This is your time to be alone with yourself; a time for you and only you. The time to do an activity as simple as walking around the block, taking the stairs and going up and down or just going to the gym for a swim in the pool or a ride on the stationary bike. This also is a good time to socialize and meet new friends. Take a daily walk and call it your "morning or afternoon constitutional" and do some stretching as you walk. On the next page, there are some balancing and stretching strength movement exercises that are divided into two forms; the silhouette or shadowy forms are for the more senior member or the less mobile adults and the colorful one's are for the more robust agile senior members. Try them all and perform these balancing and stretching strength movement exercises with a family member or friend. Pick the upright or standing exercise to improve balance and strength control, as well as, coordination. Focus on the legs muscle movements more and the twisting movements and please do these movements slowly with very little strain and in moderation. It took you years to get in the condition you are in today so now let's reverse this cycle of time to your benefit. Enjoy and benefits from these illustration.

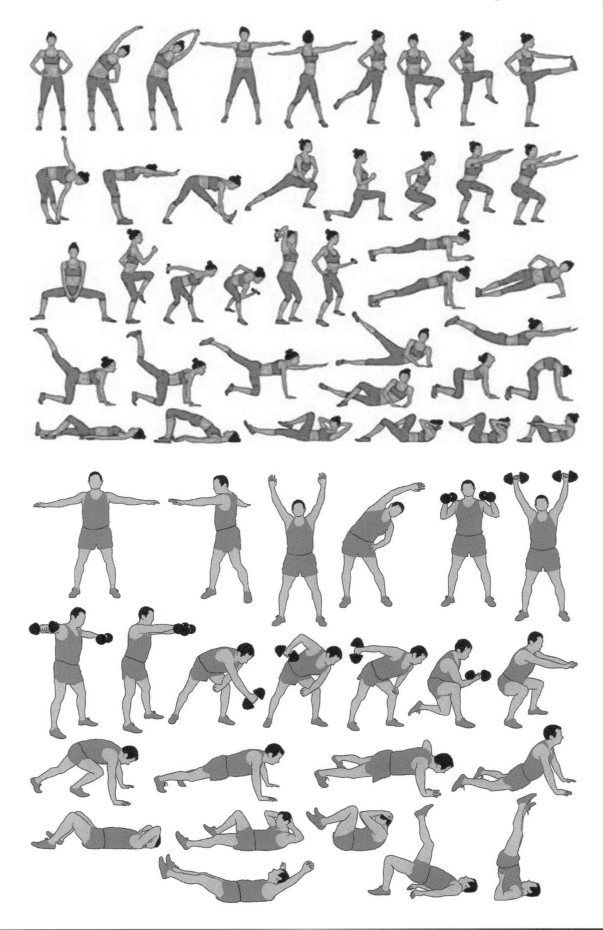

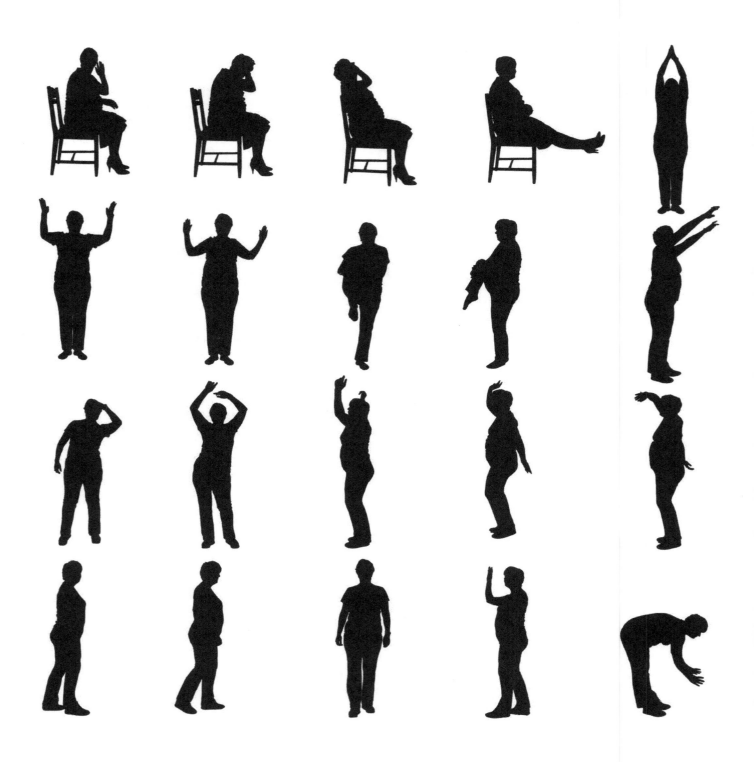

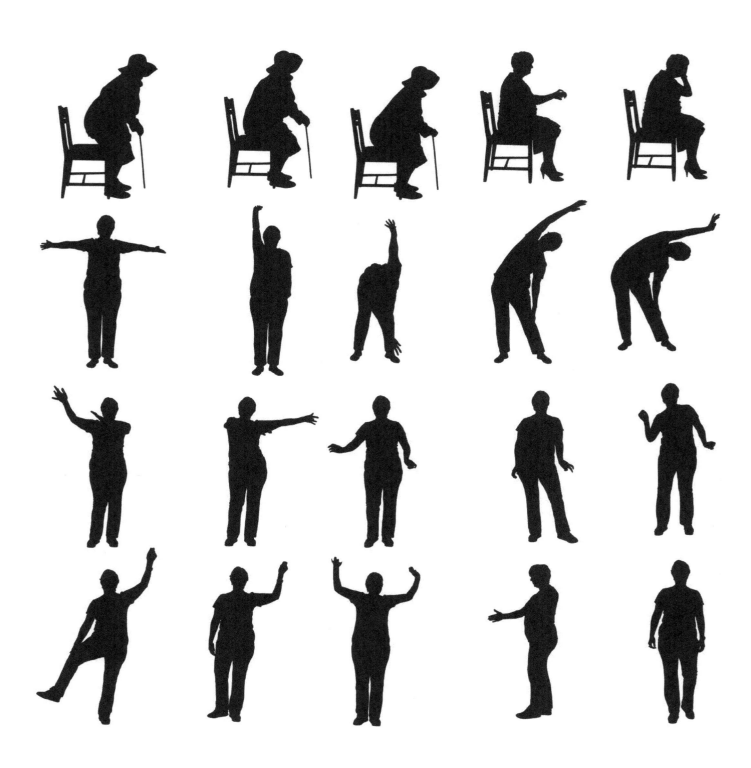

Chapter 13

Elder Injuries and Safety Precautions

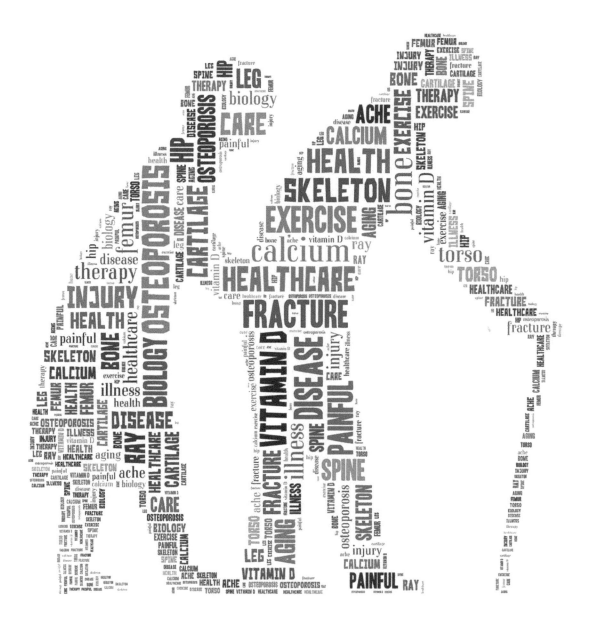

Contents in Chapter 13

Elder Injuries and Safety Precautions

The majority of Injuries are preventable but some health conditions are either new, still developing, unknown or undiagnosed. There is no blue book to follow on getting old. The most important concern is to try and prevent the most obvious occurrences of fall potentialities in keeping yourself and your love-one safe. Faith in God and in His immeasurable wisdom may have other plans for us. It is important to know some of the most common injuries that are sustained by older adults and in lieu of all the preventive measures you may take that will significantly help reduce the risk factor of falls for you and your elder love one, there is always that if. Some of the injuries that we will be covering are brittle bone disease, hip fractures, ankle and wrist sprains and fractures, and head trauma. Realizing that some of the information in this chapter may be a little stressful for you and your love one to read and to see, it is still important for you and your caregiver and other professional staff to understand them.

Brittle Bone Disease (BBD)

A person inherits brittle bone disease and there is a 50 percent chance that his/her offspring will inherit the same genetic trait. It is a life-long genetic disorder that causes your bones to break very easily even without any falls. Brittle bone disease is also called **osteogenesis imperfecta, Ekman-Lobstein syndrome or Vrolik syndrome** and it can develop in all races and hits men and women evenly. The degree of brittle bone disease is determined by what gene is affected. Some people with this condition have a bluish tint to their eyes and in some cases, deafness is one of the symptoms. As of this time, there is no known cure for this disease. The cause of the defect is that your genes do not make enough of the substance called **collagen** which is a protein that forms to strengthen the bones structure. There are many types of this disease that range in severity and degrees. The BBD that develop during fetus typically result in death within a few weeks. The prognosis for those that have a milder form of the condition and who receive good medical management and treatment is much better and many can live an average lifespan. Fall safety precautions is a critical measure with these individuals.

Hip Fractures in the Older Adult

Age is a key risk factor when it comes to hip fracture and these hip fractures actually start at the early age of 50. Hip fractures become more prevalent as one becomes older and the primary culprit is imbalance. This is usually accompanied, in most cases, with the help of poor bone mass conditions, such as **osteopenia or osteoporosis** but this can also happen with healthy bones depending on the force and/or height when the hip collides with a solid object. According to "Medical X Press" dated June 4, 2018, and I quote:

> "One in three adults age 50 and over dies within 12 months of suffering a hip fracture. Older adults have a five-to eight times higher risk of dying within the first three months of hip fracture compared to those without a hip fracture. This increase risk of death remained for almost ten years."

Osteogenesis Imperfecta

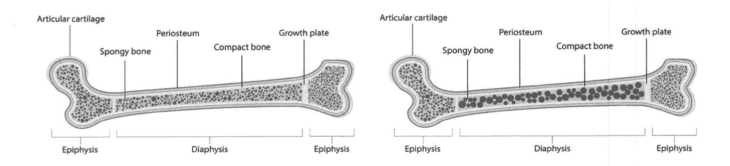

Osteoporosis

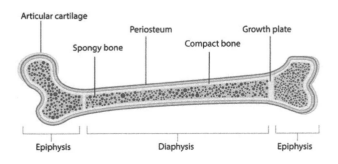

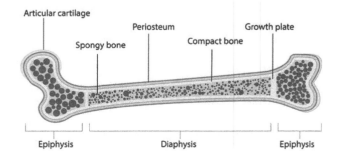

This is an alarming statistic. We are all aware of the seriousness of any fractures especially in those in the senior members of our society but to put it in the category of life-threatening poses grave concern. This is why it is so important to learn all that one can about fall preventive measures. First, what does a hip fracture refer to; well it refers to a fracture that is closest to the hip joint, such as, a femoral head fracture or intertrochanteric fracture or subtrochanteric fracture or any fracture that is closest to the ball-and-socket section of the hip where the hip moves and allows the legs to swing forward. The possible risk factors or precipitating causes of fracture are also important to understand. Balance has been discussed already so let's break down two words osteopenia and osteoporosis.

Osteopenia is a condition in which the bones have low-bone mass or low bone density. This means that the bone does not have enough minerals to maintain the bone's strength, **mass or density (BMD)**. This condition develops early in life and there is no known single cause of osteopenia. Those with a family history of this condition should have yearly screening via **DXA scanner** (specialized x-ray device for density) that may detect this condition as early as possible. Those individuals that have osteopenia have a high percentage of developing osteoporosis.

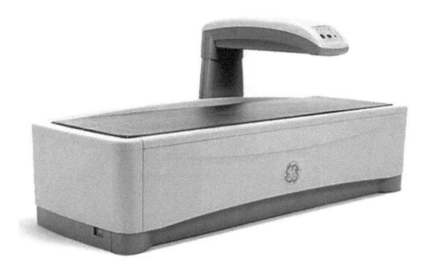

Duel-energy X-ray Absorptiometry (DXA) Scanner

Osteoporosis is the most common reason for fracture injuries due to falls in the older population and it is a disease that weakens all the bones in the body. Until there is a broken bone, there is no real sign or symptom of this condition. Bone injuries can occur in any part of the body's bony framework be it the hips, the vertebra, the wrists and ankles, and the forearms. Osteoporosis literally means porous bones and is due to the reduced density and quality of the bones. The bones continue to become less dense, porous, and fragile until the risk of fracture occurs.

Why does this happen is still a mystery. One should be mindful to understand that the bones are living and growing tissue that requires nourishment such as proteins, minerals, and vitamins just like the other body cells. Vitamin D helps the absorption of calcium and phosphorus; protein is an important building block for bones. Collagen is a protein for the knitting together of all these minerals that is important for health of the skin, hair, nails, teeth and gums, muscles and tendons, and the bones and much more.

Types of Hip Fractures

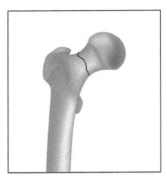

Transcervical neck fracture

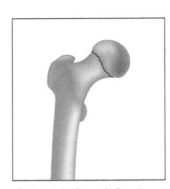

Subcapital neck fracture

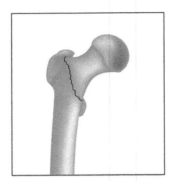

Intertrochanteric fracture

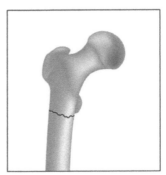

Subtrochanteric fracture

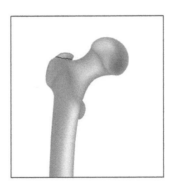

Fracture of the greater trochanter

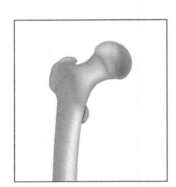

Fracture of the lesser trochanter

Hip Fracture

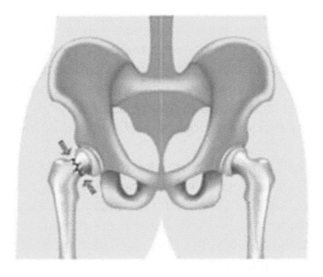

The bones are made up of the protein collagen. Collagen is a crucial factor in the mesh, hardening, and the strengthening of the bones and its framework in the body. Collagen and calcium which is 99 percent in all bones and in the teeth and, by the way, other minerals make the bones strong and help it to withstand functional use and stress. Older bones cells are removed and newer bone cells are added to the bony framework throughout one's lifetime. Bones become stronger and harder as we grow older and maximum bone strength hardness develops around the age of 20 until adsorption exceeds bone formation. In women, there is greater bone loss at the start of menopause and this continues throughout the postmenopausal years. Women are more affected by osteoporosis then men but it does affect men as well.

Risk Factors of Osteoporosis

Individuals that are more likely to develop osteoporosis disease are those with risk factors but this does not mean that those without risk factors can not develop this disease. Here are some risk factors that can be changed and some that cannot be changed:

> - **Sex** – greater in women then in men.
> - **Age** – as you become older, your bones become thinner and weaker.
> - **Body size** – small thin frame women are at higher risk.
> - **Ethnicity** – Whites and Asian women are at highest risk; African and Hispanic women are at lower risk.
> - **Family history** – family history is a key factor of fractures and those affected may have reduced density/mass and can be at high risk.

Risk factors that can be changed that are linked to falls have been discussed already.

Ankle and Wrist Injuries in the Older Adults

Ankle fractures are the third most common injuries in the older population. Hip and distal radius fractures are the first two. Most ankle fractures in the elderly patient are treated in a very conservative manner, but treatment has been found to increase mortality. Now older patients have become operative candidates and this is due to the great geriatric-orthopedic advancements in the hip fracture management of patients. In considering injuries to the ankle, we will be looking at the elder individuals 65 years and older. Doctors all recommend that one should remain as active as possible, especially in your later years. Maintaining an active lifestyle requires some physical activity but this can also have a downside. Injuries to the achilleas tendon are very common in the older population. Other injuries are pain in the back of the heal, bruises of the ankle, and bursitis. Ankle fracture injuries for older adults are more challenging and difficult to treat and with a long healing process which can lead to further complications. Risk factors like, obesity, diabetes, cardiovascular complications, and other chronic conditions can add to a longer healing possibility. It has been studied and found through duel-energy X-Ray absorptiometry (DEXA) scan that bone mineral density measuring examinations on ankle fractures was not because of low mineral density but an increase in weight and this may have had an increase probability as a risk or causative factor.

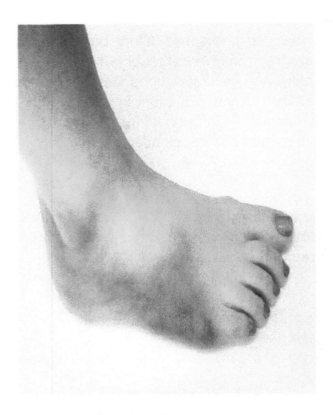

Bruised Ankle

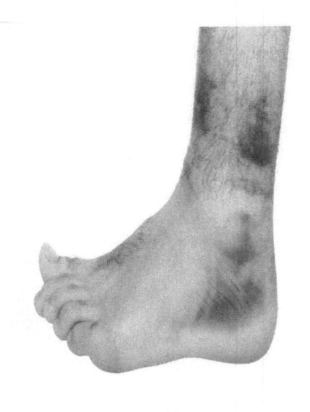

Ankle Sprain

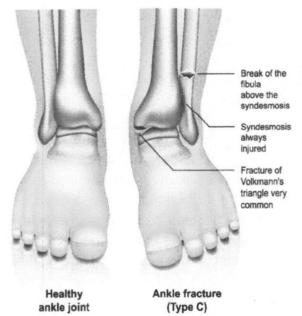

Break of the fibula above the syndesmosis

Syndesmosis always injured

Fracture of Volkmann's triangle very common

Healthy ankle joint

Ankle fracture (Type C)

Types of Ankle Fractures

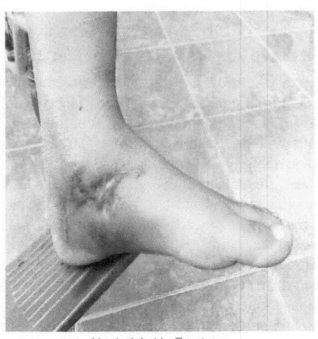

Healed Ankle Fracture

Wrist fractures are breaks or cracks in one of the many bones in the wrist. Most of the time it happens when one is trying to control a stumble or prevent a fall and, in this attempt, to catch oneself from this possible or actual fall by landing on one's hands or outstretched arms and hands. Injuries in the elderly are usually **distal radial fractures** and this is caused by trying to protect and catch oneself that is mainly due to difficulties in managing one's balance. Fractures to the wrist are usually caused by a low energy fall which basically means falls from a standing or sitting position. According to Science Daily News, one-sixth of all wrist fractures in the U.S. emergency departments are wrist fractures, 15 percent are women 50 years old or older with the majority of the falls being falls in a standing position. The studies continue to state that there was no precipitating traumatic cause or event of the fall and the fall was because of a compromised balance episode. The study continued to find that "older adults who sustain wrist fractures are more likely to have poor balance control issues then those who have never sustained any fall related injury." It goes on to state that these older adults should be evaluated and tested for balance deficit disorders to try and decrease the risk factor of possibly sustaining other falls. There are also varying severities of wrist injuries and fractures and some of the signs and symptoms and a few illustrations may help separate a sprain from a fracture are listed, but if in doubt see a doctor:

1. Pain and swelling in the wrist
2. Inability or difficulty in using the hand or the wrist
3. A deformity at the site of the wrist
4. Pain upon finger movement
5. Numbness or tingling of the fingers

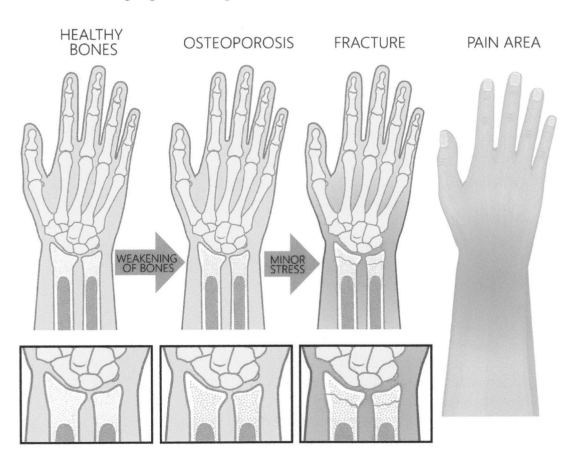

HEALTHY BONES   OSTEOPOROSIS   FRACTURE   PAIN AREA

WEAKENING OF BONES

MINOR STRESS

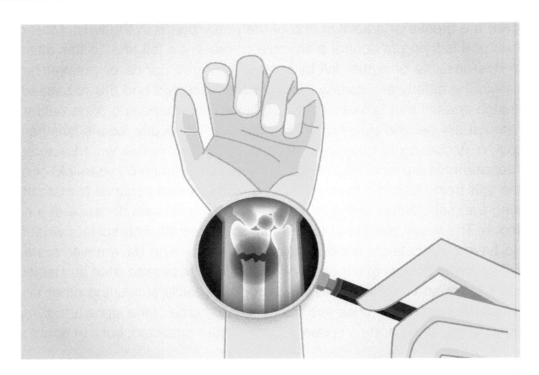

Distal Radial Fracture – This is the most common hand injury in the older adult falls

Many times, a fall by a senior adult will or can result in other injuries, such as, hip or head injuries, even a possible concussion. While balance and mobility problems are the leading causes, there may be other reasons for the fall like a physical limitation as a lower body weakness, vision impairment, and other major contributing situations. Realizing that this has been repeated throughout this script, it is worth repeating. Balance and physical limitations as low body weakness can be worked on with the senior if they would participate in low impact exercises program three to four times a week. Exercise in the pool is a great way to develop balance and leg muscle strength. Participating with light weight training, walking, Yoga, and just being socially active is a good means of moving about. It is the sedentary lifestyle that is mainly the culprit we have to fight. Take a walk – NOW!

Head Injuries/Trauma

Although head injuries in itself are serious for all ages, head injuries are more frequent in the older adult due to their risk factors. The CDC has reported that 56,000 seniors are hospitalized each year due to the result of head injuries and that 8,000 have died from these head injury falls. Head injuries that are seen in the emergency room are classified as **"traumatic brain injuries" (TBI)** which basically means any indirect force that jolts the brain violently within the skull vault where the brain shifts forcefully forward and or backwards against the boney skull **(coup and contrecoup).** This violent force can come from being struck on the head, falling on the head or sudden stop as in a motor vehicle crash. Depending on the state of consciousness and damage to the head determines the severity of the head injury. Brain trauma classification will depend on nerve damage and this can range from mild, moderate or severe and if the injury caused loss of consciousness and how long did the unconsciousness last. If the head injury is not life-threatening, that is, mild or even moderate, it can still pose a long-lasting effect on the person's cognitive function. Traumatic brain injuries:

✓ May be long-lasting or even permanent.
✓ Can include unconsciousness, inability to recall events, confusion, speaking or remembering problems.
✓ Unsteady gait (walking), lack of coordination, and problems with vision or hearing.
✓ Certain types of traumatic brain injuries may cause dementia or Alzheimer's disease.

Some signs of head injuries;

1. Changes in size of pupils,
2. Clear or bloody fluid draining from the nose or ears,
3. Bruising on the face and/or around the eyes,
4. Trouble with hearing, smelling, tasting or vision changes,
5. Irritability,
6. Lightheadedness,
7. Loss of consciousness,
8. Low breathing rate.

Any one that has a hard impact injury to the head and experiences any signs listed above should contact their doctor or seek medical attention immediately. Head injuries can become worse so, in a nutshell, it is important to have this injury followed up frequently.

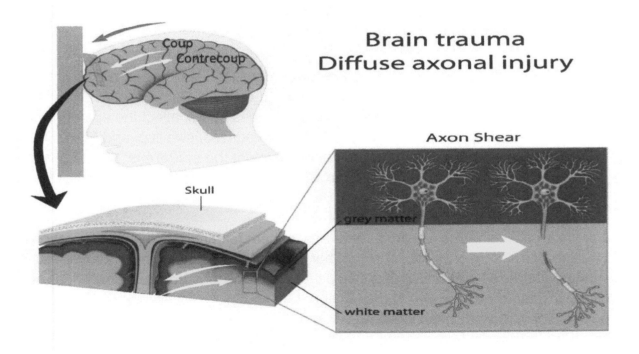

Burn Accidents

Burns, although not considered a common injury in the older population in the U.S., they are among the most common injuries worldwide and much more common in under developed countries. For the elder population, burns can be a hard injury in regard to healing because most have compromising conditions already. Older people suffer more frequently from burns because they are more vulnerable to them given their compromised mobility, coordination, and balance. These compromising conditions can also be because of other health issues ranging from heart ailments, respiratory complications, diabetes or kidney disease, mild tremors, to other difficult medical conditions which will impede the healing process especially when it comes to burns. Many seniors live independently by themselves due to death of spouse or divorces placing them at a higher risk of accidental injuries. Burn injuries can be from clothing catching fire, scalding hot water or hot grease from a stove, by cigarette smoking, and electrical burns or heater mishaps.

Recognizing the risk factors with older adults are the same as with all the elder risk factors especially those that smoke or have mini-tremors which may be accompanied by reduced sensitivity to pain. Cooking may become a hazard and may cause injuries by the elder touching the hot stove or hot pan not realizing it is still hot. **Peripheral neuropathy** (reduced sensitivity) can result in the senior not even realizing that he/she has been burned until it is too late. As we age, the skin thins, the elasticity is gone, and there is less fat at the subcutaneous layer which can lead to more severe and deeper types of burns. The classification of burns is first-degree, second-degree and third-degree burns:

- **First-degree burns** are considered mild compared to the other burns resulting in pain and reddening of the epidermis or outer layer of the skin. Sun burn.
- **Second-degree burns** also called partial thickness burns, affect the epidermis and the dermis or lower layers of the skin causing pain, redness, swelling, and blistering.
- **Third-degree burns** or full thickness burns, affect the epidermis, the dermis and the deeper layers of the skin resulting in white or blackened and charred skin that may be numb.

Some of the causes of burns are dry heat (fire), wet heat (steam or hot water), radiation or sun lamp, friction burns from a scrape or a rub, hot objects, the sun, electricity, or chemicals. The most common burns occur from what is called thermal burns that are caused by house fires, car accidents, accidents that happen in the kitchen, and electrical failures. Treatment depends on the specific type of burns sustained. Mild burns or first-degree burns are treated with skin care products like aloe vera cream and/or an antibiotic cream and for pain Tylenol. Burns that are in the second-degree range are treated with antibiotic cream and other medication prescribed by your physician. The more serious burns in the third-degree range may require more aggressive treatment, such as, grafting and intensive care intervention, antibiotics therapy via intravenous (IV) administration as well as fluid replacement therapy. As stated, burn care can be the most intense and prolonged care especially the pain management care treatment that is due and the extensive treatment needed for proper healing.

SKIN BURN

EPIDERMIS

DERMA

FAT

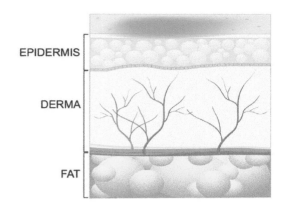

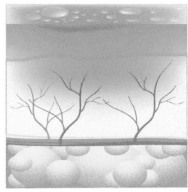

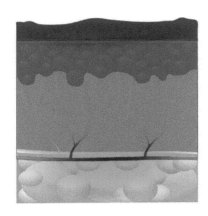

First-degree
burn

Second-degree
burn

Third-degree
burn

Chapter 14

Hospital Emergency Room Medicine and the Elder Patient

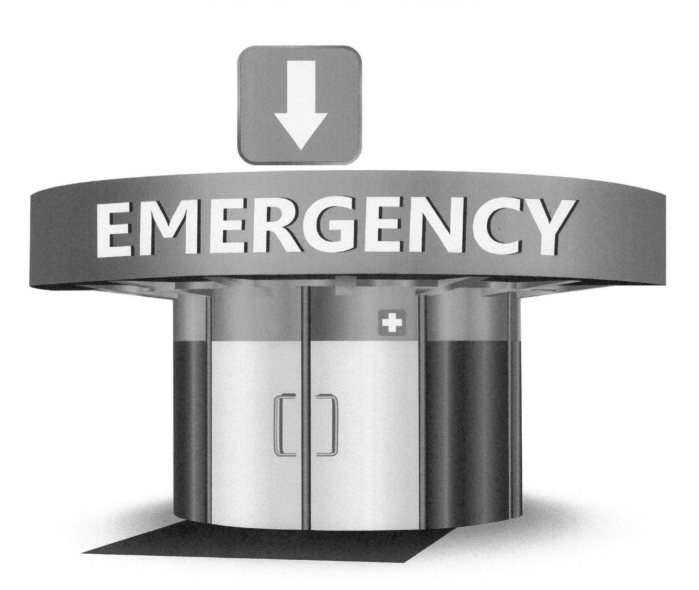

Contents in Chapter 14

Hospital Emergency Room Medicine and the Elder Patient

There has been a marked increase in the number of older adults seeking help in the hospital setting. Approximately 15 percent and as high as 20 percent of the hospital visits and/or in-house population are seniors 65 years old and over and they represent the most rapidly growing hospital residents in need of care. In fact, within the last decade the elder population visits to the emergency room has increased more than 34 percent and it is quite clear as to why this is happening. Older adults have been coming into the emergency room (ER) with a myriad of medical problems and with serious complaints such as fall injuries, dyspnea, chest pains, and abdominal pain, as well as, other complaints such as weakness, fatigue, and dizziness which may indicate more serious problems as head injuries and strokes. Compared to the younger person, older adults have more diagnostic tests done, longer waiting periods in the emergency rooms, and are the most likely to be admitted to the hospital. Although this increase is very evident in the emergency room arrivals, the elder population still seem to have more problems excessing the emergency room service. It is becoming rather clear that no one seems to really know what is an emergency and what is not and when to access immediate emergency care but at the same time, this is causing unnecessary delay and this delay means further harm to the patient. Rapid and quality emergency response depends on the value of awareness and time the service is received. Many elder adults and their love one's hesitate to call 911 for an ambulance transport service to the emergency room. Knowing the ins-and-outs of what constitutes an emergency care need may not be as clear or obvious to some as it is to others so they wait until it is physically or critically too late to make that response in a timely manner. Then there are these caregivers that would transport the older person in need of care in their private vehicle thinking that it is faster. Yes, it may be but there is a deferent protocol for personal in private vehicles verse those coming to the emergency room by emergency transport. Individuals transported by ambulance are seen immediately where as those transported by individual vehicles may have to sit in the waiting room where there will be a delay in seeing a doctor.

Family members and healthcare providers should plan ahead before the need of the ambulance service and the emergency room visit is at hand. There are certain preparations that your love-ones and/or caregiver should be doing to prepare for an eventual emergency room visit. The patient should have a list of all medications he/she is taking: dates, time, doctor's name, important addresses as well as phone numbers, any medical condition the patient has or has had, any surgical procedures the patient has had in the pass, any allergies, insurance information and legal documentation should be easily accessible to the family member or caregiver. The legal documentation should have information that have the living will or power of attorney or any other legal request made by the patient. A copy of this information can be on the refrigerator or in plain sight in the house/apartment. It would be prudent to have a "Go-to-Bag" with items that one would need in the event of an admission. Please keep in mind that the average length of time in an emergency room waiting area can be very lengthy and this ER time is on the rise. One can wait literately many hours before being seen. It is important to try and reduce stress by bringing some reading material or some form of distraction for this waiting room stress time. Keep in mind that if you, the caregiver and/or love-one become emotional, agitated or nervous this will not be good for the one you are caring for.

EMS Transportation to the Hospital

Before calling for an ambulance for yourself or your love-one, compose yourself and take a deep breath. Try to collect your thoughts and put things into perspective as to what you must do. Things can be very confusing at this time so remember the planning that you have put into play and remember the list of medications, doctor/s, names, and other valuable information to take with you as well as your Go-to-Bag. Know the number to call for emergency services and when the operator answers, give her/him the details, follow the operator's responses and answer their questions: What is the emergency - Where do you live - What is your name - What is your phone number. DO NOT HANG UP! The operator will stay on the line until the first emergency responders arrive so stay on the phone until the operator tells you to hang-up. If you are a family member, friend or caregiver, there are times when the operator may give you advice on how to help the injured person before the first responders arrive. The fact that you knew the emergency number in your area is a lifesaver and is a critical part of accessing quick response to medical services. Depending on which country you live in, the emergency access number may be different but the common thread is that they will more than likely be emergency numbers that are a three-digit figures. When the EMS arrive, give them the information that is important to the emergency situation and then other valuable information as the EMT requests it and later the other documentation for the patient. Here are some emergency numbers in different countries:

- Dial 911 (U.S. and Canada)
- Dial 999 (UK)
- Dial 000 (Australia)
- Dial 112 (Europe)
- Dial 119 (Japan)
- For other countries look up the number when you arrive in that country.

There are times when you may have to move an injured patient out of the line of further threat, or stop a severe bleeding situation and/or intercede with the patient's present condition to prevent loss of life. Only do so if this does not further endanger the patient's life or your life. If you are licensed and/or certified to perform CPR and this maneuver is needed, please do so. If the injury happens as a result of a criminal act, a police officer will be sent so please follow their expressed directions. Injuries that have occurred because of a fire or car accident, give aide until told to stop by an EMT or a police officer and follow their directions as they control the scene with the firefighters that were sent to your location as well. In all cases of injury and while the EMT or paramedics are dealing with the injured person, the police will want to talk to you and ask you questions about what you saw or what happened and/or transpired at the scene. Give them your utmost attention and answer their questions to the best of your ability.

Elder Patient in the Emergency Room

The management and care for these seniors in the emergency room is high and the status-quo for care is hard to meet and at this time, the staffing is no-longer-sufficient in most emergency rooms to meet these hospital demands and as needed. Most emergency rooms are not physically designed and prepared to handle this increase in older adult care. Staffing in emergency rooms with specialized training in senior psycho-physiological care for the older adults with their variant needs are not always there and the staff may not be able to cope with this growing trend. Many hospitals have instituted a separate senior wing section in the emergency room for this express purpose of caring for and management of this growing increase of emergency visits and needs by the elder population. In this way, they can better care for and treat the high flow of the

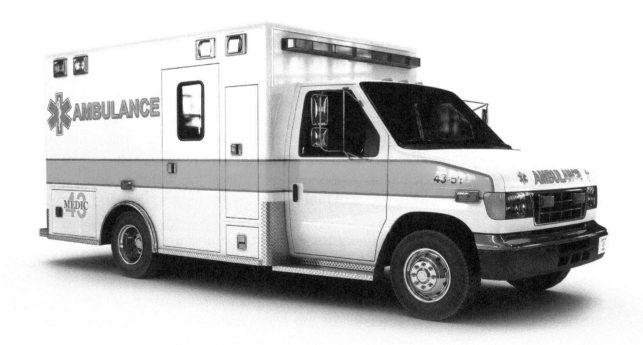

older adults and their needs as well as improve the service given to the patient. Once seniors are brought to this wing, nurses with specialized training in health issues related to the elder patients, can make assessments and determinations according to the patient's health needs and status, be it, mental and/or physical function care. Working in conjunction with other medical personal as well as social services and pharmacy staff, they will collaborate and decide on the best course of treatment modality needed based on the overall team's assessment of the entire mind-body condition of the senior patient. This is a new trend and not all hospitals have yet adopted this concept.

Elder Patient Focus Process

The senior care wing of the emergency room is basically the same as the normal emergency room. There is a triage nurse that determines the medical needs and problems related to the patient's visit and makes a pre-assessment need care protocol according to the severity of the elder's health emergency; those that qualify for immediate admittance are admitted without delay. Those patients that are in need of immediate care are brought to the senior care wing and are attended to by the nurse specialist and the medical team and a more comprehensive assessment is done. The medical staff in the senior care wing will focus solely on health issues and will determine in a holistic manner the proper approach of treatment and caring for the patient and to prevent as much as possible, the elder in having to make further hospital visits. This is why it is important for the medical staff to have all the information on the patient's medical history. The previous health history plus the ER assessment will help prevent errors in providing immediate care for the patient and to ensure that nothing will be missed and that adequate and professional care for the patient will be made and given. Many of the elder population often present with uncharacteristic symptoms such as, angina with or without pain, infections that do not have a fever or may not have an elevated white blood count, that is why having these specialized collaborative teams support working together can make the difference between life-saving care and can help and do more for the patient. They are able to handle a host of many different and chronic conditions and make diagnosis that will better benefit and serve the well-being of the elder patient. It is in this way that the collaborative team effort does its best work.

There will be many stresses during your decision on transporting your love-one to the emergency room. It is not like just dropping them off at the "ER Admission Area" and letting the hospital staff take over. Older adults need help in navigating through the morass of admission procedures and through the recording and admission phase. Throughout this time, you will experience tension, you and your love-one will be going through many different emotional amplifications that can heighten sensitive feelings and alter the state and symptoms of confusion. It is easy for others to say to you, relax, stay calm, but it is up to you to think through the situation and work through this problem smartly. Remember the protocol that has been set-up and proceed from there.

1) Be clear with the ambulance attendant and the staff in the emergency room. Tell them what happened and what your love-one medical problem is as well as any other special needs.
2) If your love-one is admitted or needs to go to another inter-departmental area, transports in the hospital can be very stressful for the older patient and this is when other more serious problems can occur. Ask the staff to be especially careful when they move your love-one from one department to another.
3) Make sure that you have the up-to-date comprehensive list of all the medications, medical procedures, etc. that is part of the elder's history. This is why it is important to make an inventory of the procedures before an emergency event occurs.
4) It is important to make sure the emergency room doctor has the entire medical history. This will prevent unnecessary medication or treatment errors.

Hospitalized Older Adult

It is very difficult to hear from your emergency room doctor that your love-one will have to be admitted. Hospitals are lifesaving institutions and if this is what it will take to help your love-one, then so be it. Thank God for the doctors and staff that have recognized this need for your love-one's admission. For the patient, it presents a form of disability, a taken away of certain freedoms, and a loss of independence. It is at this juncture when it becomes the responsibility of hospital staff to care for and to make sure that your love-one, now called the patient, maintains and continues his/her activities of daily living (ADL), receives the prescribed medication, and receives proper nutrition. The staff have a systemic approach, protocols, and plans of care for the well-being of the patients on their wards following the doctor's recommendations and prescriptions. Elder care is assessed as to their needs and their decision-making capacities and together recommendations are made. The capacity of the patient is determined by the ability to understand and communicate choices, understand questions presented, being able to present sound reasoning, and demonstrate an intellectual understanding to the present state of affair as it stands now. There are other staff members available to assess and assist in this process including social worker's and psychiatrist when there is evidence of need or depression that is, to determine the patient's states of awareness if this complication arises. Decisive treatment and then this follows management plans are made for the patient. Much of this can be obtained through the personal records brought in with the patient. You as a member of the family or a healthcare provider or even a good friend can act as the patient's advocate and monitor the medical treatment and care that is being given or provided by the staff for the patient during a hospital stay. Hospitals and the hospital medical staff only want the best for their patients but hospitals are not without their own risk factors so it is behooving on the patient advocates, love-ones and friends to support the medical staff and observe conditions that need reporting such as;

➢ Changes in mental status of the patient, especially with those 65 and older,

➢ If a patient has problems moving or positioning themself, he/she is at risk for bed sores, so be aware of this when you visit and check for bedsores,

➢ Find out the times the doctors and specialist are attending your patient. Be there if possible and in this way, you will be better informed as to what care and treatment and future care is needed or being given or done,

➢ Know the previous medications your patient was taking as well as the new medication your love-one is taking and if they are causing any side-effects,

➢ Older adults are at risk for falls, so ask questions about the medications and if they will cause side effects such as sedation, disorientation, or imbalance for your patient,

➢ Is your patient able to eat by him or herself and if not find out if he/she is being fed. Older patients in hospitals have had problems in eating and without proper nutrients recovery can be very slow,

➢ There is something called nosocomial or hospital acquired diseases such as, Methicillin-Resistant Staphylococcus Aureus (MRSA) and pneumonia that can make healing of diseases much more resistant and harder to treat so it is up to the caregiver and family member to watch for signs and symptoms of fever.

Avoiding a Return to the Hospital

It has been stated and written that older adults over 65 years of age are more likely, after being discharged from the hospital, to be readmitted to the hospital within 30 days after being discharged. Many older adults with selected medical conditions may safely go to alternative hospitalization facilities for continuing quality medical care but many other patients after being discharge are readmitted to the hospital for preexisting conditions or linked infections. These infections were presumably treated at the hospital and the patient was discharged either from the emergency room or from admission status. This has happened more frequently when patients are discharged to their homes or to a home care facility and does not usually happen when the patient is discharged to a skilled nursing home. Transitioning and discharging patients that are frail and are discharged from a hospital to a primary or long-term care setting can greatly decrease the readmission and increase the well-being and improvement of the health of the patient. Long-term care facilities are not immune to receiving patients that were discharged from the hospital that still have infections but these facilities are adept at treating these infections at their site. The best way to prevent your love-ones from being readmitted is to be a strong advocate while the patient is still in the hospital; ask many questions and don't stop until the patient is discharged from the hospital.

A. Be sure to understand all the instructions and recommendations given by your healthcare provider. The hospital's discharge personal will give you a sheet with your discharge instructions on it, read it, ask questions, and keep it hand.

B. Most patients are so glad to be getting out of the hospital that they fail to ask important questions or have an answer to a question clarified. Older patients are in a rush to get home because they may fear that their home may be gone. Family members and friends can check in on their apartment or home and take care of their pet/s and this should reassure the patients.

C. Your doctor may recommend a follow-up consultant and/or care manager or other services needed at home. Follow through with their recommendation.

D. Many patients tell their doctor that they are fine just so they can be discharged from the hospital quickly even though they may still be experiencing symptoms. This is one way to be sure that you will be readmitted back to the hospital in short order. Be honest with your doctor and prevent readmission.

It is important that the discharged patient make an appointment with their primary physician after leaving the hospital. This means a face-to-face visit and not a phone call meeting. Keep all follow up appointments; this is one of the biggest reasons why patients are readmitted to the hospital. Transportation can be arranged and provided by your doctor's staff, caregiver or friends. They can accompany you in the doctor's office and take notes for later reference. One of the more confusing parts of a discharge planning guideline is when your doctor has prescribed multiple medications, especially if you have been diagnosed with serious health issues and the medication is essential for maintaining your health status quo. Seniors may need a caregiver to help with managing and organizing home medication regiment affairs so that the patient knows how and when to take their medication. They can also check for medication reactions such as dizziness, drowsiness, increase in sleeping. Your caregiver should also monitor any changes in the senior's appetite and diet, level of pain, any change in mood such as depression, if your love-one had surgery, check the site of surgery for swelling, redness, fowl swell, or discharge from the area. Even though all of this checking, observing, and care for your love-one at home is to avoid the need for readmission to the hospital, if conditions have become so severe, please do not hesitate in bringing your love-one back to the hospital for evaluation, treatment, and if necessary readmission.

Chapter 15

Rehabilitation Therapy and its Effects

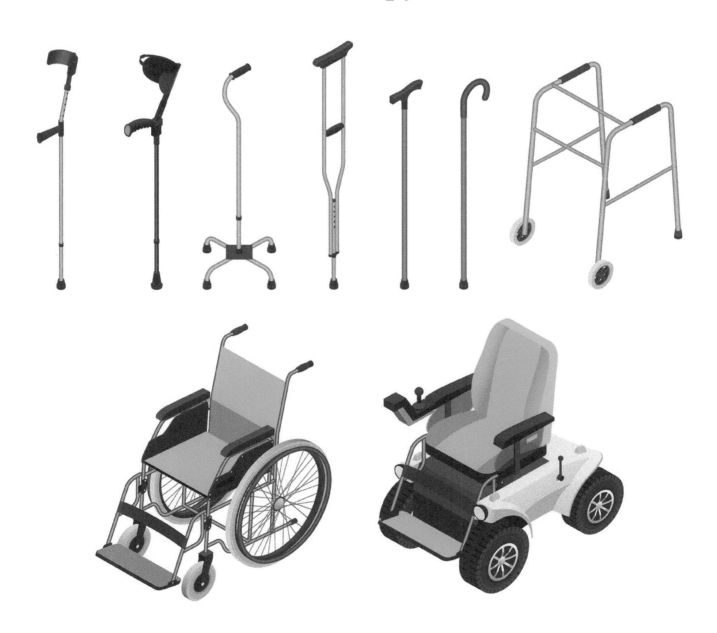

Contents in Chapter 15

Rehabilitation and its Effects

The quality of life can be greatly increased and the readmission to the hospital greatly reduced by the effective use of therapeutic techniques. Physical therapy is a great motivator and it literary gets people up and about helping people to walk and to regaining their balance. This all helps in preventing falls and reducing the need of readmission to the hospital. Physical activity and the recommended exercises can help to increase the independence and safety of seniors which can lessen the likelihood of reinjury with the added increase in the quality of life for the senior adult. There are basically three types of therapeutic follow-ups that your doctor may recommend: physical therapy, occupational therapy, and speech therapy. Your doctor may prescribe skilled nursing services for those that need a more comprehensive therapeutic modality, especially if you have wounds that are slow to heal or not healing well, edema and swelling of the limbs that are slow to reduce and return to normal, long term I.V. therapy, and other medical needs that must be attended to. Your doctor may feel that specific nutritional needs may also require follow-up and he/she may prescribe a dietitian as part of your follow up protocol. This will be by a licensed nutritionist to ensure that you are able to sustain your nutritional needs. These specific health conditions can follow illnesses such as heart failure or diabetes and a multitude of other medical complications that need a good diet regiment.

As you can see, physical therapy can be a means of returning to full independence. Physical therapy is also known as physiotherapy and is collectively called rehabilitation which can help in many daily task conditions that affect the younger and the elder population. These conditions can be from Alzheimer's to fractures to urinary incontinence to speech therapy. The geriatric section of the American Physical Therapy Association (APTA) stated that the main thing that brings older people to the physical therapist is a fall. These falls are usually after hospital admissions for a fracture, surgical treatment, and discharge planning with part of the discharge planning being a follow-up protocol treatment plan and referral to a certified and appropriate therapist. Rehabilitation is necessary and physical therapy is required to help restore strength and balance as well as range-of-motion, flexibility, coordination, and endurance while helping to reduce pain and retain and educate bruised or injured muscles. Stroke patients have a myriad of impaired physical functions, such as, loss of speech, inability to move their right leg and/or right arm but after months of physiotherapy they will be able to function again with the help from the therapist and the right attitude from the patient. In regard to speech, they will be able to communicate and regain much of their speech qualities. It has to be a shared recovery responsibility from therapist and the patient in an effort to be successful.

In the United States, older adults make up the majority of the participants in physical therapy programs, in fact, in all forms of rehabilitation programs. The major two diagnosis for the rehabilitation therapy programs is for strokes and hip fractures but there are many older adults that enter into therapy to seek help and treatment for areas other than the loss of physical function but for cognitive or mental and emotional issues. Those that enter the program with recent on-set of physical or mental problems seem to benefit the most from the rehabilitation therapy. The majority of these older patients are discharged from the hospital and some of these patients may have referrals from their hospital or primary physician to see a psychiatrist or psychotherapist, speech therapist or an occupational therapist. These are all forms of rehabilitation specialists that can help in the management of different human disorders and return the person back to his/her self-image and self-independence.

Goal of Rehabilitation for Older Adults

The general goal in rehabilitation for the older patient is to improve mobility and self-care without the assistance of any second party person. This can be determined by assessing the ability of the patient to function in the manner in which he/she performed before the occurrence of the physical or emotional medical problem. The best way to achieve this goal is through the coordinated rehabilitation of the entire multidisciplinary team of health care professionals to include nurses, caregivers, pharmacy personal, and doctors working in sync to effectively care for the patient. When it comes to falls, one of the major goals is maintaining balance and control and it is the number one predictor of elder accidents. Studies have shown that impaired ability in balancing during or while performing a task may be the result of motor and/or cognitive impairment of the brain's positional sensors which are mainly controlled by the eye positional sensors and the semicircular canals of the ear positional sensors or both to the older adult which will precipitate a fall. Ear infections can cause this imbalance and can be treated. Other positional problems and how to handle this cognitive or motor impairment glitches is still to be found. Balance related to gait, speed of gait, possibility of a falls, sensory combination miss-matches, and the ability to perform a task while standing will be assessed after weekly rehabilitation sessions. This combined with home training tasks, strength training, endurance training, controlling center of gravity training, sensory training, and posture training will all be assessed and done with significant improvement in all these measures including balance, and gait ability. It was found that rehabilitation for balance improved greatly but for dual-task ability it did not increase to the same extent. To me, it depends on what dual-task is being performed and the extent of cognition and understanding of the task being proposed.

It is important to add that many elder individuals, as they walk, especially in the sidewalks, look down at their feet when they are walking. This should not be done. Your eyes are in a direct link to your brain and the fluid in the semicircular canals as well as the saccule and the utricle which all maintain the equilibrium of the position of the body are following the directional gaze of your eyes. This information is being transmitted to the brain for geo-synchronization. The brain only perceives what is sent and all that the brain understands is this DOWN direction so, where do you think your body wants to go. It is important to try and keep your eyes straight ahead and use your peripheral downward gaze to check the ground or sidewalk. Likewise, to help maintain equilibrium, walk with a wider stance for better walking control. This may take time and practice to accomplish and get use of doing but it is much safer than the alternative. Again, please choose solid, secured, and comfortable supportive shoes to walk in.

Stages of Physical Therapy – Rehabilitation

The primary stages of physiotherapy rehabilitation should be to control pain and inflammation and to protect the injured site so that it can heal properly. There are more than fifty therapeutic approaches but only a few of them are commonly known but we will stay with physical therapy, speech therapy, and occupational therapy. What should follow from these three are the range of motion, degree, speed, endurance, torque level, and strength movements with progression of exercise integrity. There are basically four phases or stages to rehabilitation. This follows the model that best provides for the patient's needs, progression, and outcome.

Phase I – This is the early stage of the rehabilitation program when you address and control the pain and swelling factors (ice, stop aggravating movement patterns when possible, NSAIDs (pain control medication), ultrasound, electric stimulation). It is the time to relieve the immediate problem that occurs from the injury and damaged tissue.

Phase II – Once the inflammation has diminished it is time to apply some stress and mobility through range of motion and flexibility with some joint movement and possible soft tissue stretching. Early strength training may be possible but this decision is between the therapist and the patient to determine.

Phase III – At this stage range of motion has improved or is nearly back to normal and edema and swelling are gone or no longer a problem. Muscle strength and endurance is coming back, **proprioception** is functioning, and agility is close to being within normal limits. Phase111 usually begins with strength exercises and high repetitions with low resistance and continues to evolve from this point. Exercises become more aggressive in strength and muscle endurance after this point.

Phase IV – In this stage the only real condition lies with the patient. This phase mimics all the stresses that the patient will be going through when he/she returns to normal activities. This phase is to restore strength and endurance to normal or near normal planes. Flexibilities and strength activities are now at maintenance levels.

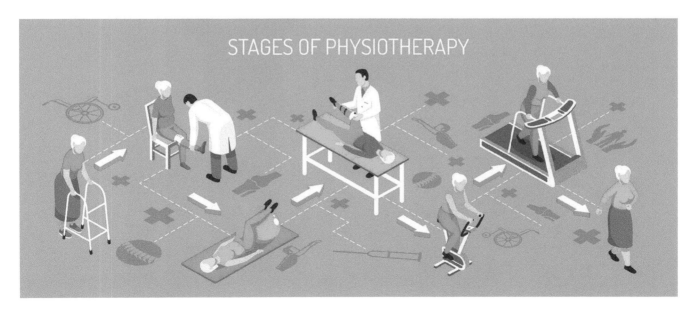

STAGES OF PHYSIOTHERAPY

The Most Common Types of Therapies and Their Purposes

Physical Therapy (PT) – As written, physical therapist provides a more physical and functional service to restore and improve mobility, reduce and relieve pain, and to prevent or limit further physical disabilities in patients with injuries and illnesses without the use of invasive methods. It treats all kinds of injuries and its purpose is to restore function to the body, maintain that function, and to restore and promote overall wellbeing, fitness and health to the body.

Occupational Therapy (OT) – The purpose of OT is to help increase the patient's functional independence in preforming their daily activities of living (ADL) and to minimize the disabilities imposed by injuries or a disease process. OT is usually combined with physical therapy and other treatment modalities to ensure uniformity of care. This type of therapy focuses on helping those with physical, sensory, or cognitive frailties to make the individual more independent in their daily lives such as eating, bathing, showering, toileting hygiene, dressing, and sexual activity.

Speech Therapy (ST) – This is a field of therapy that specializes in speech related pathology and language problems. It assesses and treats oral communication disorders and is performed by a speech-language pathologist (SLPs) which are often referred to as speech therapist. Much of this therapy involves children and young adults but since this book is about the older population, we will concentrate on them. The goal of a speech therapist for the senior is to increase oral and/or functional communication to include hand and sign language, cognitive skills, and teaching safety measures in swallowing. Speech therapy may include introductions in diet, medications, and special feeding techniques, as well as muscle retraining in swallowing with other strategies used for communication skills and trachea care devices. Speech therapy for seniors is often necessary when the patient is recovering from a disability such as a stroke or dementia and even a severe head trauma injury. Communication is important at any age but for seniors it becomes vital.

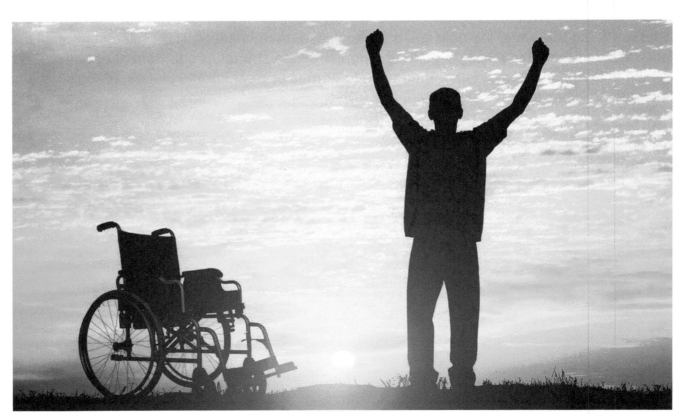

Chapter 16

Future Trends in Elder Care

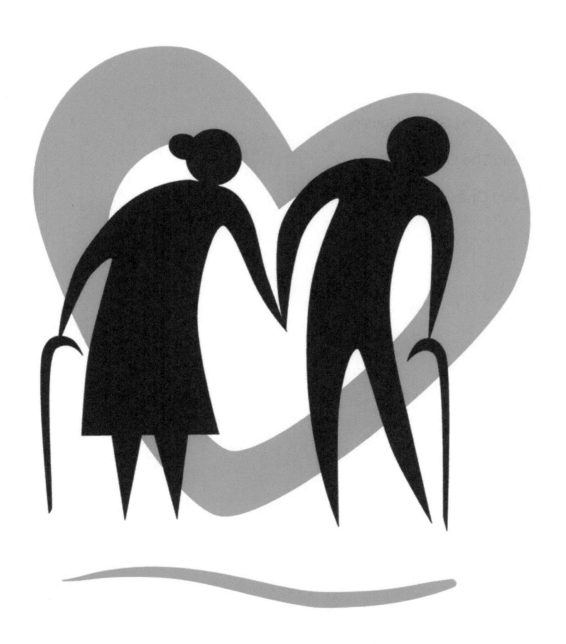

Contents in Chapter 16

Future Trends in Elder Care

According to Demographic Changes and the Aging Population there are over 45 million U.S. citizens living today that are 65 years of age and older. As time goes by, this number is expected to increase by 90 million by the year 2050. From 2020 to 2030, 18 million more Americans age 65 and older will be added to this census list which would mean that 1 in every 5 Americans will be 65 years old and over. This information was obtained by Rural Health Information Hub (info@ ruralhealthinfo.org) and this is closely compatible to the statistics in the "Population Reference Bureau's – Population Bulletin *"Aging in the United States,"* and this growth will continue as research scientists find newer and better ways to extend human life. This growth in the elder population is said to be a trend that was-and-or-is driven by the baby boom generation that may have started as early as the 1920s not only in America but throughout the world. Staying just in American the elder population trend demographics, we have passed through many stages of the baby boomer generations and drifts so to better understand these stages I have clarified them here. As you will probably see, each generation follows a general yearly pattern which basically means when one generation passes the other will fill the void;

The Silent Generation are the people born before that of the baby boomers around the mid-1920s to mid-1940s,

The Baby Boomers generation are those born between the early 1940s to the early 1960s.

The Generation X are considered those born between or about 1966s to 1980s,

The Millennial generation range from the early 1980s to the early 2000s,

The Generation Z is the name of the children after the Millennials that were born later in the 1990s and early 2000s,

The Xennial Generation are a blend of two words between Generation X and Millennials and it is meant to describe a micro-generation also called a cross-over generation of people whose birth years are between the late 1970s and the early to mid-1980s.

I am sure that history will put the next and the next and next decade of Americans in a nice fancy and catchy generation word phase criteria as above to explain histories future breaks in the age population time gaps.

Fluctuation in Population Growth

Throughout the many years of mankind's existence, we have managed to increase our life expectancy. The most commonly used measure for measuring life expectancy is the **Life Expectancy at Birth (LEB)** method which is the mean length of time of an organism's average life based on the year of birth to the year of death. This measurement takes into account many demographics as well as gender and compares them to those born decades ago when all members have died. The National and World LEB figures report that in the Bronze age and the Iron age, the LEB was 26 years. Coming close to present times and going world-wide the LEB in 2010 was 67.2 years, in Eswatini (Swaziland) it was about 49 years, and in Japan the average age was 83. In the U.S. in 2020 the life expectancy is about 78.93 for males adding five more years for females. What may be surprising to some Americans is that we are not the highest in this life expectancy at birth to death category. According to the United Nations projection World Health Census for LEB, Hong Kong is the highest at 84.89, Japan is 84.67. Macao 84.30, Switzerland 83,84, and the United States is pretty low on this list down around 39 of the LEB range. This LEB statistics fluctuates in that one decade it will be high 78.93 and the next decade it may drop to around 78.64. LEB goes both ways depending on the country or certain events be it environmental, disease as in the flu or coronavirus, it can also be a manmade event such as military conflict. The coronavirus pandemic of 2020 will definitely influence and probably lower the life expectancy at birth rate throughout the world from the 2020s to 2030s or another decade to follow. It is important to put into some prospective that in the U.S. there is a continuous diversity in the population increase and decrease in the composition of its growth. This compositional also changes in its racial and ethnic groups that fill the gaps in each generation. It is also important to understand that in America older adults are staying in the workforce longer and this goes for both genders. As stated in previous chapters, this age chronological stereotyping and using 65 as the determination stereo criteria of old age, will have to change due to this massive increase in the aging life's expectation.

Scientist will continue its research life's potentials and to try and extend the life expectancies of the human race in search of the holy grail; to seek the ream of immortality but until that time we will have to except the role we play in this short expectation ream of life which basically is the present longevity prospects.

Growth of The Aging Population

There are a number of good developments that have transpired for the older population in the health field and health technology that have improved the needs of this demographics. Much of these improvements are designed to be useful to the older population such as smartphones, home technology, voice first hardware as in virtual assistance, and in-home sensors. These devices will help the older adult and their caregiver improve their health, safety, and quality of life. This is especially important today when it comes to those that have the functional ability and are mentally capable of living in their homes and in their community. Age should not be a factor if the older adult has the physical and mental capabilities to manage his/her own affairs and environment. There are a number of important aspects in this **"Aging in Place"** viewpoint that must be considered and these are economics, access to transportation, the accessibility for their love ones and of their caregivers to communicate and commute to them geographically to care for them. It is also important for the care receiver to understand this expected supervisory arrangement role and to accept this care proviso. As the population of Americans continues to rise and as long as there are caregivers and love ones willing to take on this responsibility, as well as, having the government's attention and support and is prepared to accept its role in this type of care, it would be a service to all to encourage this trend of Aging in Place.

In most parts of the world older family adult members live in the same household of their families or relatives and are cared for by family members but in America there are much less older family members that live and stay in the same family nucleus. This may be a prearranged decision or that their parents are not wanted in the immediate family circle. Circumstances may play a role in this family nucleus for instance social, economic, or living space being inadequate. Whatever the reason, some parents will more than likely live on their own and/or with their spouse or partner. In the U.S. and in other countries with advance prosperity, economies, and with higher education standards, the family nucleus tends to have fewer children and you would think that they should help support their parents in their homes. This is not the case. Most older adults in America are in adult care facilities which are many and varies in care and treatment modalities. This may be by the senior members own choice and/or decision or lack of choice due to medical or mental conditions. Many countries have cultural and religious reasons for keeping family members together and others countries may find it more affordable for older people to stay in their own home. The percentage or rate of the older population living alone in many European countries are much higher than they are in the U.S.

Aging in Place "Yes or No"?

According to the research done with **"Home Instead Senior Care, Inc.,"** seniors have overwhelmingly chosen the desire to age at home. This does not mean that seniors want to stay in the same home in which they have raised their families, but to live in a new home that have newer features and more conveniences within and without their new home. Some of these seniors are willing to invest in these amenities for these added accommodations. Those that want to remain in their own home would like to see age-friendly modifications made to their present living conditions to make it much more convenient and safer. When it becomes a decision maker or choice that has to be made to these seniors, it can become deeply personal and emotional with strong desires by the senior to stay at home. The senior will express a fear of loneliness or their fear of becoming isolated which is what happens in most cases then not, this may impact their decision matrix. Whichever the case, seniors want to remain as independent as possible and this can be heartbreaking to love ones that have a senior that cannot physically and/or mentally care for himself or herself on his/her own. Safety of the elder love one must, must take precedence.

Older Americans and Senior Housing

In a Harvard Joint Center on Housing Studies (JCHS) for _Housing Americas Older Adults,_ they write that our graying Americans need more affordable and diverse housing developments for renters and owners. The article goes on to suggest that this "tsunami of older Americans is just starting to crest;" and that these present households will have older members in their family nucleus that will be 70, 80, and 90 years of age due to this baby boomer generation growth potentiality. Housing worries will prevail and become scarce and that there will not be adequate housing and other services for the middle-income population as this graying of Americans growth potential continues. The need for more affordable housing will become crucial and there is an immediate need to shift to providing homes and rental options as well as building senior housing in urban centers and safe walkable suburbs with numerous lifestyle features in good neighborhoods. Technology should be a part of the new developing projects. Those with means are moving to other areas and congregating in senior living communities, such as, North Carolina, Michigan, Oregon, and parts of California, to mention a few geographic regions. Those that lack the means end up Aging in Place and some of these areas they do not have adequate medical services and social services to care for this rising growth of older adults. The housing of the very low-income seniors has decreased and will continue to decrease as the aging population rises. Housing and Urban Development.Org. (HUD) is aware of this challenge and the need to increase this housing burden for seniors and it is one of the hallmarks of their pressing responsibilities. There is a large wealth disparage between today's retired population but as more baby boomers age, there is going to be an overall financial decrease which means that the household will be unable to generate the same level of wealth for retirement due to this growing and pressing needs. There are some solutions such as increasing subsidies and low-income units, modifying homes with assistive devices that can make Aging in Place better and safer. This can help in keeping seniors at home and happy rather then sending them to assistive living facilities funded by Medicaid. We must find a way to get in front of the growing need.

Technology and The Older Adult

Technology among older adults is becoming the new trend and is growing. Seniors are drawn to this new trend and are learning to use smartphones, smart speakers, and home technology such as the phone talk feature, computers and iPads, navigate through smart TV using the streaming online and other options to watch shows, and many other voice assistant smart devices according to AARPs National Survey. The purchase of technological products by older Americans is now 51 percent and rising and the research by Brittne Nelson Kakulla of AARPs survey done January 2020 indicates that the growth rate is just going to go higher by our senior Americans. At present the percentage is:

- Smartphone 23%
- Computer and laptop 12%
- Smart television 11%
- Tablets 10%
- Smart home technology or device 12%
- Wearable devices 7%

Through their family or on their own, many older adults have installed home safety technology devices such as video cameras inside and/or outside their apartment or homes. Some have installed sensors that monitor windows and doors for safety and peace of mind. This peace of mind and safety is not the same when it comes to understanding the internet though. It seems that trouble appears when it comes to online information. The elderly tend to divulge more information online then they should or believe in too much information online as fact. Accepting too much information that is received on the internet can reprehensibly cause family damage and financial devastation. The confidentiality, privacy, and safety of any and all information placed on the networks can never be guaranteed and that goes for any and all smart devices.

In the U.S. alone only 7.5 percent of the younger population have used voice assisted devices for healthcare reasons, such as, Alexa or Google in 2019. Many healthcare workers, at least 52 percent would like to use it if they had the opportunity to help them in their patient care service and 45 to 60-year-olds are more optimistic and hopeful about having and learning to use this technology for their healthcare related service. When talking about voice assisted technology, we're talking about smartphones, smart speakers, and other smart voice assisted devices such as Apple Siri, Google Assistance, Samsung Bixby, and their ability to support and give aide to healthcare users in cases of need. It is also noted that more older Americans 60 and up are on the tablets, computers, and smart TVs and spend a lot of time on these devices. This rise is seen in both genders and it does not matter the education levels of the elder. Indeed, this trend is spreading towards more mobile technology and online services. When talking about the elder population we're talking about all racial and ethnic groups, in fact, one quarter of the Hispanics and one quarter of the blacks share and use smartphones as their internet provider compared with one-in-ten whites. The use of other smart devices like laptops and desktop computers are actually going down. Beyond the age criteria, there is a distinct difference how smartphones are used when it comes to educational levels of the user for instance higher educated older adults use the internet via the cellphone whereas college graduates mostly use their computers to go online. This may be the result of household income, race, and ethnicity or just plain convenience. The smartphone has become such an asset to older adults that they credit their smartphone as to why they have not subscribed to a higher-speed home internet service.

Protect My Love One

As much as we do not want to think about it most of our older population will end up in a nursing home. This will be our love one's and/or our final destination. Choosing the proper nursing home or assisted living facility or an in-home medical care plan can become very complicated and often is a very emotional time in our lives when a hard decision has to be made. This decision will take a very strong disposition in each of us to entrust our love ones to the care of others and sometimes this trust is not reciprocal with the one's that you have given this trusted to care for your love one. Senior citizens are abused and neglected in some of the best nursing homes or assisted living facilities. These frail and vulnerable love ones may not be able to express or help themselves and depend on others to help them meet their daily needs. The aides, nurses, doctors, and administrative staff have the responsibility to meet these needs and to care for these elderly more vulnerable patients and protect them from harm. This is not always the case.

Residents of these facilities may and do sustain injuries, are neglected, become dehydrated, are malnourished or develop infections and/or bedsores. Some sustain non-intentional physical injuries or by intent by staff members mishandling the patient or just plain physical abuse and assaults to patients. The use of restraints can be over used or the forgetful nurse may neglect to put up the siderails on the bed if there is a need to put them up. Neglect can also come from emotional or oral threats to the patient and if this is happening to one patient it may be happening to other patients. All staff members, including the dietitian workers and cleaning staff, have a duty and a responsibility to report any and all such abuse.

Every State in our Great Nation have laws against elder abuse be it in a nursing home or at your home, on the streets, or anywhere and if it is observed it must be reported to the proper authorities. There are laws protecting you and the older adults from being exploited and physically or mentally abused. This abuse can also come in the form of financial and personal mishandling. In the nursing home it is up to the nursing staff to identify this abuse and report this abuse to the doctor and administrative staff immediately but this does not always happen. Family members and patient advocates discovering this abuse themselves should report this abuse to the nurse, doctors, and administrative staff. An investigation is to be undertaken immediately by the facility and remedies are to be forthcoming to resolve this matter at the nursing level. It is also important that this be reported to your attorney so that an outside investigation can be done as soon as possible. There is a time span on these types of cases so do your due- diligence without delay. It was truly an honor and a pleasure writing this book. God bless you and your love ones.

At this point I will say thank you for your time in reading this book and I hope it was of some help to you and those in which you are caring for – Thank you.

Glossary

A

Abiogenesis – is the informal name for the origin of life on earth from the non-living matter to an organic compound.

Adiponectin – is a specific protein that has been said plays a role in the development of insulin resistance and atherosclerosis. It circulates in high concentrations in the lean person but in obese subjects it is much lower.

Aerobic – related to, or involving, or requiring oxygen.

Adenosine Triphosphate – is the main molecular energy for all cells in the human body and is made up of adenosine molecule and attached to 3 phosphate groups.

Aldosterone – is a steroid hormone produced by the zona glomerulosa of the adrenal cortex in the adrenal gland. Its purpose is to conserver sodium in the kidney, salivary glands, sweet glands, and in the colon. It maintains homeostatic regulation between the B/P, plasma sodium (Na+) and potassium (K+) levels in the human body.

Anabolism – is the process which the body utilizes the energy release by catabolism to synthesize complex molecules. There complex molecules are than utilized to form cellular structures that are formed from small simple precursors that act like building blocks.

Anaerobic – related to, or involving, or an absence of free oxygen.

Apoptosis – is the death of cells which occurs as a normal and controlled part of an organism's growth or development.

Arteriosclerosis – is the thickening and hardening of the walls of the arteries, occurring typically in the elderly.

Asprosin – is a protein hormone produced by mammals in the white adipose tissues that stimulate the liver to release glucose into the bloodstream.

Atherosclerosis – is a particular type of arteriosclerosis, but term are sometimes used interchangeable. Atherosclerosis is the building up of fats, cholesterol and other substances in the and on your arteries.

Atrophy – is the partial or complete wasting away of a part of the body.

B

Baroreceptors – are located in the carotid sinus and the aortic arch. Their function is to sense pressure changes by responding to change in the tension of the arterial wall. The baroreflex mechanism is a fast response to change in blood pressure.

C

Catabolism – any destructive process by which complex substances are converted by living cells into simple compounds, with release of energy.

Chemical bond – is a lasting attraction between atoms, ions or molecules that enable the formation of chemical compounds.

Chemical reaction – occurs when two or more atoms bond together to form molecules, or when bonded atoms are broken apart.

Cloning – is the process of producing generically identical individuals of an organism either by natural or artificial means.

Codicil – is an amendment to a Will; a Will that modifies or partially revokes an existing or earlier Will.

Cortisol – is a steroid hormone of the glucocorticoid class and produced in many animals' tissues in low quantities. It is released with diurnal cycles (circadian rhythm) and released in response to stress and low blood glucose concentrations.

Coup and contrecoup – is an injury to the brain that occurs in the front of the frontal lobe region or front of the brain (coup) and the back of the brain occipital lobe or back of the brain (contrecoup). This basically implies that there has been a traumatic injury to the brain causing a contusion/bruise of the brain tissue. Coup means blow)

D

Deoxyribonucleic acid – is a molecule composed of two chains that coils around each other to form a double helix carrying the genetic instructions used in the growth, development, functioning, and reproduction of all known living organisms and many viruses.

Diploe – is the spongy cancellous bone separating the inner and outer layers of the cortical bone of the skull?

Duel-energy X-ray absorptiometry (DXA) – is a means of measuring bone mineral density (BMD). Two X-ray beams with different energy levels are aimed at the patient's bones. When the soft tissue absorption is subtracted out, the BMD can be determined from the adsorption of each beam by bone.

E

Element – is a substance that whose atoms all have the same number of protons.

Endogenous – a chemical or substance that originates internally.

Eukaryote – are organisms whose cells have a nucleus enclosed within membranes.

F

Frailty – a condition of being weak and delicate especially in the elderly.

Free Radical – are a chemical species that contain a single unpaired electron in its outer orbit.

G

Genetic – related to or determined by its origin, development, or causal antecedents of something.

Genealogy – an account of the descent of a person, family, or group from an ancestor or from older forms.

Genome – is an organism complete with a set of DNA, including all of its genes. Each genome contains all of the information needed to build and maintain that organism. In humans, a copy of the entire genome, more the 3 billion DNA based pairs, is contained in every cell that has a nucleus.

Genotype – the genetic makeup, as distinguished from the physical appearance, of an organism or a group of organisms.

Geriatric – related to old people, especially in regard to their health care.

Gerontology – the comprehensive multidisciplinary study of aging and older adults.

H

HeLa cells – is an immortal cell line used in research. It is the oldest and most commonly used human cell line. The line was derived from the cervical cancer cells taken on February 8, 1951 from Henrietta Lacks, a patient who died of cancer on October 4, 1951.

Homeostasis – the tendency toward a relatively stable equilibrium between interdependent elements, especially as it pertains to maintaining the physiological processes.

I

Inherent Parens Patriae – is Latin for parent of the fatherland/nation. In law it refers to the public policy power of the state to intervene against an abusive or negligent parent, legal guardian, informal caregiver, and to act like the parent of any child or individual who is in need of protection.

L

Lipofuscin – is the name given to fine yellow-brown pigment granules composed of lipids and contain residues of lysosomal digestion. It is considered to be one of the aging or "wear-and-tear" pigments found in the liver, kidney, heart muscle, retina, adrenals, nerve cells, and ganglion cells. **(Also called lysosomal)**

Longevity – a long duration of an individual's life.

M

Marfan Syndrome – is a genetic disorder of the connective tissue which varies in people. It is seen usually in people that are tall, thin, long arms, legs, toes, fingers, and are very flexible and have scoliosis. Complications usually include heart and aorta disorders, such as, mitral valve prolapse and aortic aneurysms, lung, eye conditions also bone and spinal cord problems.

N

Neurodegeneration – is the progressive loss of structure or function of neurons, including death of neurons.

Neuroglia – a class od cells in the brain and spinal cord that forms a supportive structure providing homeostasis, protection, and insulation for the neurons.

Niemann-Pick Type C – is a rare and progressive genetic disorder characterized by an inability of the body to transport cholesterol and other fatty substances (lipids) inside of cells. This leads to the abnormal accumulation of these substances within the various tissues of the body including the brain tissue.

Non Compos Mentis – not sane or in one's right mind.

Nucleotides – any of several compounds that consist of a ribose or deoxyribose sugar joined to a purine or pyrimidine base and to a phosphate group and that are the basic structural unit of nucleic acid (such as RNA and DNA).

O

Orthostatic – is a form of low blood pressure that happens when standing up from a sitting or lying down. This does not have to be due to underlying disease. Dehydration, pregnancy, and anemia can precipitate this state.

Osteopenia – is generalized reduction in bone mass that is less server than that resulting from osteoporosis. It is caused by the resorption of bone at a rate that exceeds bone synthesis.

Osteoporosis – is thinning of the bones with reduction of bone mass. This is due to the depletion of calcium and bone protein. This condition predisposes a person to fractures which are often slow to heal and/or heal poorly due to this calcium deficiency.

Overload Principle – means that you have placed a greater stress load on the body than it is normally accustom to handling.

P

Peripheral Neuropathy – is a general term describing disease affecting the peripheral nerves, meaning nerves beyond the brain and spinal cord.

Phenotype – the observable properties of an organism that are produced by the interactions of the genotype and the environment.

Phospholipid – is the main component of the cell membranes, and is made up of lipids attached to a phosphate group.

Phosphorus – is a chemical element that works with oxygen to form the molecule phosphate. Phosphorus has an atomic number of 15 and is represented as a P.

Photosynthesis a process by which green plants and some other organisms use to synthesize food form carbon dioxide and water. In plants it generally involves the green pigment chlorophyll and generates oxygen as a byproduct.

Primordial Soup or Prebiotic Soup – is the hypothetical set of conditions presented of the earth around 4 – 5 billion years ago. It is the fundamental heterotrophic theory of the origin of life first postulated by Alexander Oparin and John Burdon Sanderson Haldane in the 1920s.

Proprioception – a sensory receptor which receives stimuli from within the body, especially one that responds to position and movement.

R

Ribonucleic acid – are any of various nucleic acid that contains ribose and uracil as structural components and is associated with the control of cellular chemical activities.

S

Sarcopenia – means a gradual decrease in the mass and strength of skeletal muscle tissue and a decline in mobility and quality of life due to the aging process.

Senescence – is the condition or process of deterioration with age causing loss of the cells to power and grow and divide?

Sclerosis – is abnormal hardening of the body tissue.

Secosteriods – is a type of steroid with a "broken" ring. The word **secosteroid** derives from the verb Latin: secare meaning "to cut", and Latin: stere of steroid, meaning "solid, three-dimensional". Secosteriods are alternatively described as a subclass of steroids or derived from steroids.

Senesce – a state of being old or the process of being old.

Sequela – is a pathological condition resulting from a disease, injury, therapy, or other trauma. Typically, a sequela is a chronic condition that is a complication which follows a more acute condition. It is different from, but is a consequence of, the first condition.

Specificity Principle – which is stated as the S.A.I.D. principle and most be integrated into a resistance training program so that the type of demands placed on the body and which is under your control well be adapted if done will using the F.I.T. principles.

Specific adaption to imposed demands Principle (S.A.I.D) – means if you do an exercise frequently and in good control, the body will except the extra demands you have put upon it.

Stem cells or germ cells – are cells with the potential to develop into different types of cells in the body.

Stenosis – is narrowing of the space within the vessel. This can also refer to the narrowing of the spinal space called spinal stenosis. In this condition pressure is can be exerted on the nerves that travel through the spine, especially around the neck and lower part of the spine.

Streptococcus pyogenes – is a common bacterium that causes strep throat (streptococcal pharyngitis), impetigo, other skin infections, rheumatic fever, scarlet fever, glomerulonephritis, and invasive fasciitis.

Synapse – is a structure that permits a neuron or cell to pass an electrical or chemical signal to another neuron or to the target effector cell.

T

Telomeres – is a region of repetitive sequences at each end of eukaryotic chromosomes in most eukaryotes. Its purpose is to protect the ends of the chromosome from DNA damage or from fusion with other chromosomes.

Telomerase – also called terminal transferase is a reverse transcription enzyme that carries its own RNA molecule which is used as a template when it elongates telomeres.

Thermogenesis – is the process of heat production in organisms.

Thermoregulation – the maintenance or regulation of temperature: the maintenance of a particular temperature of the living body.

Tachycardia – means a rapid heart rate that the rhythm in which the heat beats is to fast during a normal rest state.

Index